THOUGHTS
are
HABITS *too*

THOUGHTS

—— *are* ——

HABITS *too*

Master Your Triggers,
Free Yourself from Diet Culture, and
Rediscover Joyful Eating

AMY LANG

Niche Pressworks
Indianapolis, IN

THOUGHTS ARE HABITS TOO

Published by Niche Pressworks; NichePressworks.com
Indianapolis, IN

Library of Congress Control Number: 2023921130

ISBN
Hardcover: 978-1-952654-92-3
Paperback: 978-1-952654-91-6
eBook: 978-1-952654-93-0

THIS BOOK IS DEDICATED
TO MOM AND DAD

Acknowledgements

I WOULD LIKE TO acknowledge the tremendous help given to me in birthing this book. For their knowledge, wisdom, and guidance, I wish to thank Pam Ableidinger, Joyce Orsini, Toni Bauer, David McGuire, Dominic Matteo, Christine Li, Evelyn Tribole, and James Wedmore.

Also, special thanks to Nicole Gebhardt, Michael Hauge, and the rest of the Niche Pressworks team for handling this project with such a deft touch. And, of course, my abiding love and gratitude to Matt Martell for his unwavering support and uncanny ability to make me laugh.

Mostly, I am beyond grateful to my clients for inspiring me every single day.

Table of Contents

Introduction

A NOTE FROM YOUR FUTURE SELF

Dear Current Self,

Thank you so much for choosing to read Thoughts Are Habits Too. *You don't know it yet, but you are going to save so much time and energy and prevent so much frustration and disappointment with this one decision. Because of it, you'll be able to take advantage of this author's 20 years of experience in health and fitness and research to understand what it takes to achieve lasting weight loss and, more importantly...*

How to lose weight in a way that takes care of your physical health without harming your mental and emotional health.

And with the same framework Amy uses with her clients inside her coaching program, Joyful Eating Circles, you'll embrace the self-care habits and practices that make it possible to live the life you've always wanted.

By the time you finish this book, you'll know how to identify and let go of the beliefs that have gotten in the way of your happiness, and you'll be well on your way to healing your relationship with food and restoring your sense of well-being. I know because I'm you, and I've done all of this!

Remember: Love yourself. You are worth it.

Your Future Self

P.S. For a sneak peek into what's in store, take a look at the **Joyful Eating Roadmap** at ThoughtsAreHabitsToo.com/Roadmap.

Foreword

GET YOUR POWER BACK

IN THIS WONDERFUL BOOK, *Thoughts are Habits Too*, Amy Lang shares a delightful and essential guide to creating and sustaining good, healthy habits. As a friend and colleague of the talented author, I can assure you this book is a joy to read. You'll see your current self and envision your future self as you read.

Amy skillfully demonstrates the profound impact of joyful eating, loving yourself, and having mindful habits. She emphasizes the importance of making necessary shifts to create a healthy and fulfilling life.

Amy delves into the psychology and science of habit formation with clear explanations and interesting case examples. She helps us understand our own resistance and frustrations while paving the way for us to embrace her practical, doable, and effective strategies for change.

Amy's empowering frameworks — the "Fundamental Five" and the "Easy and Inevitable Method" for healthy eating and successful weight loss — foster a stronger connection between ourselves and our thoughts, decisions, and actions. She shows us how to release the weight of the judgments and opinions of others and remove the negative influences from diet culture and our past dieting experiences. She encourages us to choose our ideas and principles wisely and on purpose so we can stay authentic and loving within ourselves.

By following Amy's guidance, you can gain the power to create a life on your own terms. Strengthened, healthy, and centered in your body and mind, you can focus on what truly matters, leaving behind rigid perfectionism for personal authority and well-being.

Amy's passion for helping others shines through every word. Her heart and mind are fully engaged, ready to educate, inspire, and love in every interaction. This book is her generous gift to us all.

—Dr. Christine Li, Clinical Psychologist

Chapter 1

UNLOCK YOUR POTENTIAL

"WHEN WAS THE LAST time you were happy with your body?"

My new personal trainer, David, asked me this question during our initial meeting.

I racked my brain like I was rewinding a movie of my life, looking for an instance. I looked at him with a furrowed brow and felt a lump in the pit of my stomach.

I couldn't think of one.

I was so confused. I thought that when my previous trainer had helped me lose weight and get down to 22 percent body fat, I had figured out what it took to be happy and healthy.

Yes, I was happy that I was stronger and fitter.

And I was happy that I didn't struggle to find clothes that fit when I stood in my closet.

And I was definitely more confident in my abilities.

So much so that in 2003, I left my six-figure position in the high-tech world to become the owner of Pacific Heights Health Club in San Francisco.

Why?

Because with the rising rate of obesity in the US and the corresponding increase in chronic illnesses like hypertension, type 2 diabetes, and heart disease, I felt a calling...

A calling to be part of the solution by helping folks lose weight and get fit, so they could be stronger, healthier, and ultimately, have a higher quality of life.

But then, two months after I took over the health club, the fitness trainer I'd been working with for the past two years moved to Arizona.

I tried working out on my own, but I wasn't consistent.

"Too busy," I told myself. As a new business owner, I could easily rationalize the decision.

Plus, I really didn't like exercising by myself, and I didn't know what strength training exercises to perform or the proper sequencing.

And pretty soon, I wasn't working out at all. I was also stressed and having a hard time sleeping through the night.

As you probably guessed, my weight started creeping back up.

This wouldn't do.

I wanted to set an example for members of the health club, so with January around the corner, I decided to find a new trainer. I chose David, who had joined the team just a few months earlier.

He was the salt of the earth, but was I ready to get this vulnerable with him? After all, even though he was an independent contractor, I was technically his boss.

He asked again, "When was the last time you were happy with your body?"

"I can't think of one," I told him. Even at 22 percent body fat, I still longed to be thinner and had saved outfits I couldn't fit into yet.

"Not ever?" he prodded.

I kept searching, and then, in my mind's eye, a distinct memory from my teenage years came into focus.

It was a Friday night, and, as usual, my family was watching the TV show, *The Dukes of Hazzard*.[1] One of the characters on the show was Daisy Duke, played by Catherine Bach.

At the time, she was 25 years old and 5'8" tall, and her character often wore a short-sleeve shirt tied up to show off her cleavage and toned midriff, and cutoff shorts, which accentuated her very long, lean legs.

As she appeared on the TV screen, my dad looked over at me and pointed to her. "She has the perfect figure," he declared. Who knows why he felt compelled to do that? But it certainly did a number on my self-esteem.

At the time, I was only 14 years old and 4'11" with a somewhat stocky build. This served me well in gymnastics, but if Catherine Bach's figure was the gold standard of beauty and sex appeal, there was no way I could compete with that.

On numerous occasions, my mom also noted that her waistline was a mere 22 inches when she graduated from college. At 14, mine was already 23 inches. I felt so defeated.

Telling David about this, I added, "I can't think of a time when I haven't been self-conscious about my body. Maybe when I was 4 or 5? To this day, I know my dad is still judging it when I'm around him," I said.

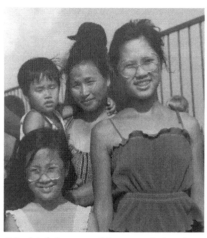

Me (right) at age 14, around the time I had this conversation with my dad.

Lucky for me, David was also a life coach. He looked at me with sympathetic eyes and asked, "I know this question is going to sound a bit odd, so bear with me," he paused for a moment. "Are you waiting for your dad to compliment you on your figure? Do you need that to feel good about your body?"

Somewhat taken aback, I replied, "Well, now that you put it that way... No, that just sounds wrong in so many ways. I'd prefer he not say anything about my body or anyone else's, for that matter."

"Okay, now that we've settled that, what do YOU need to feel good about your body?" he asked.

And with that one question, we started a process of healing.

WHAT MATTERS MOST

DAVID HELPED ME RECOGNIZE that so many of the beliefs I was operating under reflected the diet culture we are immersed in — a culture that ties your worth to the size and shape of your body and one where thinness is universally better. In addition, physical attractiveness is the currency in diet culture, so if others deem you to be more attractive, you are given higher social standing.

As we unpacked this, David asked me, "Is this what really matters to you?"

It had never occurred to me that these ideas — which I had accepted as true and internalized as the rules to live by — were not facts or laws of the universe but just opinions. Granted, a lot of people may share the same idea, but that doesn't mean it's right. A lot of people believed the earth was flat, too.

I thought about my own values, my priorities, and the kind of person I wanted to be. They had nothing to do with the number on the scale or with my figure.

Then he asked, "Why do *you* want to lose weight? Really think about what you want and why you want it."

He asked me why again and again, getting me to clarify my answers and identify what was important to me. We went five "whys" deep before it happened — a fundamental shift in my motivation and one that would define a before and after for me.

I realized that I had been chasing outcomes and focusing on what others thought of me. In other words, my first few whys were about trying to avoid the harsh criticisms of my dad, constantly comparing myself to others I thought were more physically attractive, and depending on compliments I received to feel better about myself.

It wasn't until we got to my fourth why that I discovered *the key to my health and happiness was to focus on what I thought and how my thoughts made me feel.* I wanted to BE HEALTHY. That mattered more than looking a certain way. And I wanted to get there legitimately with healthy habits.

And finally, on my fifth why, I could articulate that it was about being in integrity — keeping my word to others and myself.

In other words, what I valued mattered.

Which meant I mattered.

And not because of what I had already accomplished in life but because I was already enough.

And slowly but surely, I made more and more decisions aligned with this.

Instead of constantly asking others, "What do you think?" and seeking and relying on their validation, giving all the control of my happiness to external forces...

I started asking, "What do I want?" and giving myself permission to be true to myself.

I started paying attention to my thoughts, how I was interpreting them, and what I was making them mean — especially what I was making them mean about me.

I started noticing how these interpretations triggered the emotions that determined my actions.

I started asking better questions, like, "Because I deserve to feel good, what am I choosing to do today to take care of myself?"

And I found my actions fell into four categories: love, nourishment, trust, and gratitude.

With David's help and a lot of reflection and reframing, I also let go of thoughts that no longer served me.

And guess what?

I felt lighter. I had more energy. I made better choices. I formed new habits, and weight loss was one of the natural by-products.

These days, I call it "embracing your moxie."

I chose "moxie" because I believe real, enduring change and growth require courage, know-how, and determination.

And embracing your moxie means you're coming from a place of "I'm good enough already, I have what it takes within me, I'm worth taking care of, and I deserve all the goodness that comes from it."

When you do this, things start to flow. It's where the magic happens.

YOU ARE WHAT YOU SAY

FERNANDO FLORES IS A world-famous business consultant who uses his insights into language to transform companies and people. He did an interesting exercise at a seminar at Harvard's Cronkhite Graduate School.[2] Let's do it now.

Read the following sentence in a deep, loud, say-it-like-you-mean-it voice:

"Life seems hopeless, bleak even. I have nowhere to turn. No one to turn to. What is more ominous still is that this will never change."

(Imagine about a hundred people repeating this in unison.)

"Nothing will help. There is no one to turn to. It feels like the Almighty has forgotten me. Times are hard. They will not get better. They will probably get even worse, though this is beyond imagination."

What are you experiencing?

Is there a heaviness in your chest? Do you feel choked up? What actions are you likely to take or not take, given your current state? And will they help you reach your long-term goals?

Probably not.

Yet, chances are, some version of this dialogue has been playing over and over again inside your head, and you've been listening.

Yes, your inner critic is alive and well.

CHANGE YOUR SOUNDTRACK

WHEN YOU WAKE UP in the morning, what are the first thoughts that run through your mind? What mood do they set?

Do you feel like you slept well, or did stress, worry, and your to-do list get in the way?

What about when you stand on the scale or look in the mirror? What do you say to your reflection? Or when you look in your closet, trying to decide what outfit to wear?

Do these voices in your head fill you with confidence and empower you to be the best version of yourself, or do they leave you feeling inadequate and keep you from even showing up?

A study from 2020 puts a person's average number of thoughts at 6,200 per day.[3]

How many of your thoughts are you actually aware of? Probably a small percentage of them.

Awareness notwithstanding, they are influencing the decisions you make and the actions you take throughout your day.

Each behavior you choose is motivated by the reward or payoff you anticipate. The payoff doesn't have to be pleasurable. In fact, most of the time, we're focused on avoiding pain and discomfort.

Think about it.

What's the purpose of emotional eating?

What about saying yes when you want to say no?

Or that second glass of wine after a stressful day?

Or binge eating?

These are habits that involve taking some kind of action to avoid negative emotions.

Now, what about procrastinating?

Or overthinking, worrying, and ruminating?

It feels like you're taking action because your mind is busy playing out scenarios, but these thoughts get you nowhere.

They actually keep you from taking real action.

And after encountering the same problem a few times, your brain automates the process to save time and energy, and now you have a habit.

> **habit.** *something that you do often and regularly, sometimes without knowing that you are doing it.*[4]

Yep, just like emotional eating, late-night snacking, and scrolling on your phone, some of your thoughts turn into habits too.

And these kinds of habits can undermine your best efforts. Instead of making you happier and healthier, they're leading you toward outcomes you've been trying to avoid.

Like when you're getting dressed in the morning, and looking in the mirror brings a twinge of disgust, so you avoid social gatherings and isolate yourself to hide your shame.

Or when you don't want to buy pants that are a bigger size, so you wear the ones that are uncomfortably tight, and then you have to deal with a constant reminder of the extra fat you're carrying around, which makes you feel even worse.

Or when you find yourself snacking late at night in front of the TV, you beat yourself up, so you eat more to get some temporary relief from the pain, only to have the guilt well up even more.

It's a vicious cycle that feels impossible to break.

But that's exactly what you're going to do.

THE WAY FORWARD

IN THE FOLLOWING PAGES, I will teach you how to master your triggers so you can break old habits and form new ones.

We'll review the Fundamental Five habits for lasting weight loss and figure out which one habit you'll want to focus on first for best results.

Then, I'll share the essential practices you'll want to put in place so you can let go of the beliefs that no longer serve you, heal your relationship with food and your body — better yet, find peace and pleasure around food — and finally create the conditions that make achieving your weight-loss goals easy and inevitable.

Because life is too short not to eat the cake, drink the wine, and enjoy the company.

Note: The magic can't happen unless you apply what you learn here and practice, practice, practice... because just like swimming, you can read all the how-to books and watch all the how-to videos money can buy, but you won't actually know how to swim without getting in the water.

Start by going to **ThoughtsAreHabitsToo.com** to download and print the free roadmap and workbook. Then pour yourself a big glass of water, find yourself a comfortable chair, and prepare yourself for a fun, fulfilling transformation.

Ready?
Let's get started!

Joyful Eating Roadmap (free)
ThoughtsAreHabitsToo.com/Roadmap

Official Companion Workbook
ThoughtsAreHabitsToo.com/Bonus

IN THE BONUS, you'll find high-resolution color versions of all graphics, full versions of the exercises contained in this book, helpful worksheets, and more.

Chapter 2

DARE TO DREAM BIGGER

IF YOU'VE BEEN STUCK on the weight-loss struggle bus waiting for your stop, it's time to gather your belongings and stand up.

Because you're about to get off.

You just need to answer this question.

WHY do you want to lose weight?

When I sat down with my client Julia for her initial consultation, I asked her this exact question.

She answered matter-of-factly, "Because I'm disgusted with my body."

Her reply broke my heart. It meant when she looked in the mirror, this was what her inner critic was saying to her — like a soundtrack to a movie, setting the tone.

So... what about you? What's your why?

Is it the same reason as Julia's? Or is it another? Maybe...

- You have an upcoming event, but nothing in your closet fits right now, and you're loath to go up a size.

- You don't like the way you looked in pictures from a recent holiday gathering.

- You're tired of the aches and pains you've been tolerating.

- You don't want to have to take so many medications.

- You don't want to hear your doctor or spouse or some other well-meaning person or an online troll tell you that you need to lose weight.

- You don't want to have to ask for a seat belt extension ever again.

Whatever your answer to this question, I'd like you to pause and reflect for a moment. Think about what you are saying to yourself.

GET CLEAR ON YOUR PURPOSE

MORE OFTEN THAN NOT, the reasons why people want to lose weight are stated in terms of what they don't want. In coaching, this is called an avoidance goal.

If you're doing this, it's going to be hard to stay motivated.

Instead, try restating your why in terms of what you *do* want.

For example, instead of wanting to lose weight because you don't like the way you look in pictures, try thinking of it as wanting to love the way you look in pictures.

Do you feel a shift in the energy with this one change? Perhaps less ache and more hope?

This is still probably not enough to have the staying power needed to form the new healthy habits that make lasting weight loss inevitable.

For that to happen, you need to identify a compelling why. And you can do this by asking a series of questions that starts with this follow-up question as David did for me.

Why is it important to you?

For example, why is it important to you to like the way you look in pictures?

Do you like the way you feel when you receive compliments? Or is it more that you want to avoid the harsh judgment of others? Again, notice whether your answer is focused on avoidance — what you don't want — or approach — something you do want.

To identify a truly compelling why, we need to go even deeper.

As a matter of fact, you'll want to go five to seven levels deeper until your why generates an emotion that creates the same level of energy as the statements in the previous Fernando Flores exercise, but positive ones, filled with hope and love and possibilities.

This means it's important that you're in a positive state when you're performing this exercise. The thoughts you have, the things you say to yourself, matter.

Actually, before we continue, let's recover from the previous exercise. Please read the following sentences out loud in the same deep, powerful, say-it-like-you-mean-it voice as you did before.

Life is full of hope and possibilities. I am surrounded by friends, family, and mentors who want to help me succeed. What is even more exciting is that change and growth go hand in hand.

Say it with conviction.

I am resourceful. I am courageous. Times may get hard, but I am strong and resilient. The best days are yet to come and are beyond imagination.

In order for you to get the results you desire, it's vitally important to align your thoughts with your emotions and actions.

Because your thoughts trigger your emotions.

And your emotions are what drive your actions.

And actions, repeated over time, produce results.

When I ask my clients, especially those who are moms, "Why is this important to you?" I know I'm on the right track when I see tears start to well up.

It's a sign that they've been putting everyone else's wants and needs before their own. It's probably been a while since they've been a priority, and what's important to them has been ignored or subsumed or simply denied for a long time...

Until now.

Here's how Julia got to her compelling why.

Why #1: Why do you want to lose weight?

"Because I'm disgusted with my body."

Answer restated: "I want to feel good about the way my body looks. I want a flat tummy, toned arms, and some muscle in my upper body."

Why #2: Why does that matter?

"Because I want to be able to sit by the pool, wear a bathing suit, and not feel like I need a cover-up."

Why #3: Why is that important to you?

"Because I want to be able to sit by the pool and not worry about what other people are thinking."

Why #4: Why is that important?

"Because then it means I'm feeling good about myself, and when I'm feeling good, I'm more assertive and confident."

Why #5: Why do you want to be more assertive and confident?

"When I'm more assertive and confident, I'm willing to take risks, go after what I want — things I really care about — and I'm much better about getting together with friends and family and socializing."

Why #6: Tell me more.

"Spending time with the people I love, being there for them, it's what makes life worth living. And I want to feel like I gave it my all, that I contributed and made an impact."

WHAT YOU REALLY WANT

NOT IT'S YOUR TURN: What do you want, and why do you want it? Not what someone else wants for you or what's realistic. What do YOU want? If you want unbreakable motivation, you need to get clear on these things.

And notice that your compelling why is actually about looking at the big picture. Or you can think of it as your North Star. Let it be your guide.

Too often, when we lose sight of the big picture, we set goals that are out of sync with what truly matters to us.

For example, if you want to lose weight in order to be healthier, but then the way you go about doing so results in muscle loss, which then leads to additional weight gain and increases your risk of osteoporosis and cardiovascular disease, it's time to revisit the goal-setting process you're using.

Try this instead.

Create Your Dream Life

Again, it's important here that you feel GOOD before starting. If you feel stressed, overwhelmed, or rushed, find a better time to do this very important exercise.

What we are about to do is your crucial responsibility as the CEO of your life... because if you don't, who will?

Okay, are you in an "I feel good," James Brown kinda state? Awesome!

Let's do this!

Imagine you've achieved your goals. Perhaps it's three years from now. Or maybe it's taken less time. Maybe it's 12 months from now.

How would you describe the future version of you?

Close your eyes. I really want you to picture yourself in this moment.

What sounds do you hear? What do you smell? What do you see?

How do you feel?

What does a typical day look like? A typical week? Where are you? How do you spend your time? Whom do you spend it with? What new habits do you practice?

Now come back to the present. Write it down. Make it detailed and vivid.

This exercise is about starting with your intentions. It's about getting clear on the kind of person you want to be, how you want to live each day, and the life you want to create, and then filling in the blanks with the goals — the milestones — that let you know you're on the right track.

Now that you have a better sense of where you want to go. It's time to figure out exactly where you are now so we can plot a path to connect the dots.

(By the way, this exercise and a "Meditate on Your Joy" audio file to get you in the mood can be downloaded at ThoughtsAreHabitsToo.com/Bonus.)

START WHERE YOU ARE

BEFORE WE CONTINUE, I want you to acknowledge the great work you've done so far. It takes courage to put a stake in the ground and claim what you want.

Now you're going to need to get really honest about where you are today. No judgment. But we can't talk about weight loss or health without talking about your choices around food and eating.

We all know food isn't just fuel, as in energy or nutrients. Food is also about culture, how people express love, how we celebrate, and more.

When it comes to eating, our relationship with food — why we eat and how we feel when we eat — will determine many of the results we get. Unfortunately, for many, this relationship is fraught with challenges.

Let's take a look at five common eating personas and the frequent thoughts, feelings, and behaviors of each one.

See which one you relate to the most. Or, like astrology signs, you may be on the cusp and identify with more than one. That's perfectly normal.

The Healthy Eater. You have a healthy relationship with food, seeking out nutritious food and other activities, like exercise and sleep, to nourish your mind and body because it feels good. You do this because you love yourself and believe you are worth the effort.

You enjoy eating healthy foods and find eating pleasurable, both alone and in the company of others. You listen to your body, paying attention to when you're hungry, when you're full, when you're tired, etc., and you trust and honor what it is telling you to do. You also notice how you feel when you've taken care of yourself, and this motivates you to continue.

You're free from diet culture, having let go of beliefs that no longer serve you, experiencing no guilt when eating any kind of food.

And eating doesn't interfere with pursuing other goals in life. Rather, it enhances it.

The Intuitive Eater. You eat foods you want and like without feeling guilty. You notice things like hunger, fullness, and satisfaction when eating, and honor what your body is telling you.

You don't associate exercise with eating or weight loss. Instead, you focus on appreciating what your body can do.

You don't rely on counting calories, limiting carbs, tracking points, strict food rules, or meal plans for the sake of weight loss.

And while you've rejected the diet mentality, you are still "angry at diet culture that promotes weight loss and the lies that have led you to feel as if you were a failure every time a new diet stopped working and you gained back all of the weight," according to Evelyn Tribole and Elyse Resch in their book, *Intuitive Eating*.[5] As a result, you are still constantly triggered and upset by the media, advertising, physicians, your social media feed, and perhaps even your bathroom scale.

The Conscious Eater. You are preoccupied with food and careful about what foods you eat, often restricting foods that are deemed unhealthy, such as those made with refined sugar and flour, as well as alcohol.

You often plan your meals and snacks in advance to control portions, macros, calories, or points. You are also concerned about how food is prepared and spend a lot of time reading and scrutinizing food labels.

You also pay attention to what others are eating, often suggesting they follow your lead.

Because you are restrictive in your approach, you look forward to cheat days. At the same time, when you do eat unhealthy foods, you wind up feeling guilty.

The Unconscious Eater. You often experience extreme hunger and fullness because you either don't plan when to eat or ignore your hunger cues until you're ravenous. And then, as a result, you wind up eating too much, too fast.

When you eat, you're often multitasking instead of paying attention to the eating experience itself — as in the taste, texture, aroma, temperature, or quantity. You eat because the food is there, whether you're hungry or not.

You have a tendency to use food to solve non-hunger problems. In other words, you eat when you're not physically hungry. Eating is often a coping mechanism for boredom, stress, anger, frustration, sadness, or loneliness. Eating offers temporary relief from the discomfort of some negative emotion caused by a task you dislike or a situation that's causing you pain. And you often experience pangs of guilt for overeating.

The Fearful Eater. You experience anxiety and guilt around food — *any food* — and follow strict rules for the sole purpose of weight loss. You've been ignoring or have lost touch with the signals your body is sending regarding your hunger and fullness.

You're preoccupied with the caloric content of foods and see exercise as a way to mitigate the intake of any calories, even if you are already underweight.

You also have persistent and intrusive thoughts about what you believe are defects in your body.

Note: If you're nodding your head because this description fits you to a T, chances are, you are at high risk for developing an eating disorder. Please seek help from a qualified healthcare professional.

YOUR TRAJECTORY

IF YOU'RE A CHRONIC dieter, you're probably a combination of the Conscious Eater when you're "on a diet" and the Unconscious Eater when you're "off."

You probably don't have an eating disorder but are experiencing disordered eating because you spend a lot of time thinking about what you "should" be doing to lose weight.

You're feeling lost and frustrated, and sick and tired of being stuck on the proverbial weight-loss roller coaster — having lost weight, only to gain it back and then some — and you're desperate to get off this f*ckin' ride.

And depending on how often you've toggled back and forth between these two states and how much weight you've lost and gained each time, your chances of developing a chronic illness such as type 2 diabetes, high blood pressure, high cholesterol, and cardiovascular disease have likely increased over time.

If you continue doing what you've been doing, you are probably hoping you'll stay about the same, but the reality is you're on a trajectory (see Figure 1).

Figure 1: Your Journey Over Time

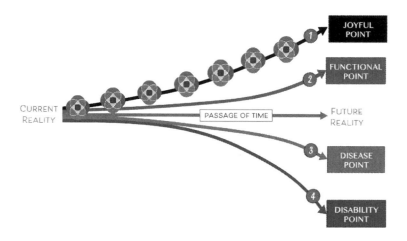

If you're a healthy eater, you're likely on line 1 or 2.

If you're an intuitive eater, you're likely on line 2 or 3.

If you're a conscious eater, you're most likely on line 2 or 3.

If you're an unconscious eater, you're most likely on line 3 or 4.

If you're a fearful eater, you're likely on line 4.

Please note: If you're on line 4 and you suspect or know you have an eating disorder, please seek a licensed healthcare professional for help. What's going on is far more complex than a book like this can address.

If you're a chronic dieter, you're probably on line 3, which means that unless something changes, you're probably going to continue overeating and weight cycling.

On top of that, between chronic diseases like high blood pressure, cardiovascular disease, and type 2 diabetes, and the back pain and knee pain from the extra weight you're carrying, you'll be taking more and more medications and be at higher risk of serious injury from falls as your physical health deteriorates.

Mentally and emotionally, your preoccupation and guilt around food, along with the body shame and self-loathing you marinate in, can also lead to isolation, mood swings, and depression.

This is no way to live, and you don't have to settle. You deserve better.

SET YOUR NEW HEADING

WHAT CAN YOU EXPECT when you become a healthy eater? How about a higher quality of life, including:

- Maintaining your optimal weight

- Freedom around food

- Feeling good about your body and yourself

- A strong, supportive network of friends and family

- Joyful eating — no guilt or anxiety, only pleasure

How much would you love to be on line 1?

Well, the way to move forward only requires you to take one tiny step at a time.

FOCUS ON WHAT YOU CAN CONTROL

TO MAKE AN EFFECTIVE course correction, instead of chasing the outcomes you want, focus on creating the conditions for them. Pay attention to the choices you're making and the actions you're taking today.

The Fundamental Five

Why are we creatures of habit? So we have the energy to focus on what matters. It's how we get important things done. Once we've automated a process, things can happen without much perceived effort.

Like the Colorado River carving out the Grand Canyon, the cumulative and compounding effect of habits cannot be overstated. Each action you choose will move you either closer to or further away from your goals.

Which leads us to these two questions: What behaviors, aka process goals, do you want to focus on? And how do you create the consistency that's most likely needed?

Here are the daily behaviors: the Fundamental Five self-care habits:

* 7–9 hours of 😴 sleep

* 1/2 your body weight in ounces of 💧 water

* 5 servings of 🥦 🍊 veggies and fruit

* Eat until you're comfortably full 😊

* 30 minutes of mindful 🏃 🤸 🧘 movement

So how the heck do you make these healthy habits stick? By focusing your attention on specific kinds of thoughts.

Scarcity vs. Abundance

When it comes to weight loss, have you tried to avoid eating "bad" carbs?

Did you do really well for a while?

And then that voice inside your head kept getting more and more insistent and telling you, "Eat that piece of pie. You know you want it. It's only one piece. C'mon... what can it hurt?"

It becomes an urge too hard to resist.

Here's what's happening.

When we try not to think of something, one part of our mind follows the instruction while another part continuously "checks in" to make sure the thought is not coming up — bringing it to mind.

In other words, if you tell yourself you can't have something you want, you are triggering a psychological state of scarcity.

And if your brain and body haven't been getting enough nutrients, you've created a physiological state of scarcity.

Either one of these makes whatever change is involved unsustainable.

This is why most diets and weight loss programs don't work.

To make habits stick, you need to learn how to shift your mind from a state of scarcity to one of abundance.

When you're in a state of scarcity, you're coming from a place of lack and fear, you see your choices as all or nothing, you're comparing yourself to others and feeling less than, and you're accepting and operating under limiting beliefs.

When you're in a state of abundance, you're coming from a place of love and acceptance, you see your choices on a continuum, you're grateful for what you have, and you believe you are enough and have enough — enough time, enough resources, and enough of what you need to achieve your goals.

Practice Detachment

One of the most common mistakes people make when it comes to setting goals is focusing on the outcomes instead of the process.

Outcomes or performance goals are things like winning a tennis match, getting hired for your dream job, finding the love of your life, or achieving your optimal weight. You don't

To make **habits stick,** you need
to learn how to **shift your mind**
from a state of scarcity to one
of **abundance.**

have control over the outcome — not without putting a thumb on the proverbial scale.

On the other hand, you can control your behaviors, such as how much you practice, how you prepare, and your attitude. In other words, you can create the conditions for greatly increasing the chances of getting the outcome you desire.

So, for the best results, focus on falling in love with the process.

The Brain's Priorities

Your brain is constantly on the lookout for threats to your survival and security in order to keep you safe — physically, mentally, and emotionally.

Just imagine if your ancestors mistook a rock for a bear. They probably would've breathed a sigh of relief, had a good laugh, and survived to live another day. However, if they mistook a bear for a rock, they would've significantly decreased their chances of passing on their genes.

Safety and security are why we prefer certainty over uncertainty... because we fear the unknown. This means any time your brain perceives that your wants and needs are at risk of not being met, *its default is to look for ways to end the uncertainty.*

It's why quick-fix solutions are so appealing.

And it's also why diets are so alluring. We're told, "Do this, and you'll get this result in x amount of time," in no uncertain terms.

Remember... a desired outcome doesn't have to be a pleasurable reward. *More often than not, the payoff is about*

*For the **best results**,*

*focus on **falling in love***

*with the **process.***

avoiding pain and discomfort — like wanting to lose weight to avoid the judgment of others.

Habits help keep you safe. Not only that, they are also incredibly efficient. That's another one of your brain's priorities — to conserve energy.

Because your ancestors had to cope with feast and famine, your brain is always looking for ways to conserve energy.

IT GETS EASIER

FORMING NEW HABITS, ESPECIALLY early on, requires intentional thought, deliberate practice, and a lot of energy.

A lot of conscious planning, problem-solving, and decision-making processes — executive functions — take place when you're applying new concepts and integrating them into your day-to-day life. The cognitive load can be huge.

Here's an example of what I mean. Think about the first time you got behind the wheel of a car and had to back out of a garage. You had to remember to do a lot of things:

- Adjust the seat

- Check the mirrors

- Put on your seatbelt

- Turn on the ignition

- Check the headlights

- Put the car in reverse

- Check for traffic and pedestrians

- Determine how much pressure to use on the gas pedal

- Decide which way to turn the steering wheel

It's a pretty long list. No wonder keeping it all straight was so nerve-racking the first time.

What about now?

Yep, old habits require a lot less conscious effort. That's why we're creatures of habit. Habits do a great job of keeping us safe and conserving energy.

But to create the life you want, growth and change are required. This means getting outside of your comfort zone. It means letting go of old habits that no longer serve you, so you can make room for new ones that do.

Again, to create the life you've always dreamed of, you'll need to:

- Know what you want and why you want it.

- Start where you are.

- Focus on what you can control.

- Put your trust in the power of habits.

- Recognize when you're in a state of scarcity vs abundance.

Now let's take a closer look at your triggers.

Chapter 3

UNCOVER YOUR LIMITING BELIEFS

WHEN WAS THE LAST time you were triggered? What's your go-to way of coping? Do you meditate, go for a run, or are you more like Tina Fey in the *Saturday Night Live* skit after the 2016 election, when she was gorging on sheet cake?[6]

When it comes to mastering your triggers, it's helpful to look at the bigger picture. Take an inventory. Look at ALL of your habits — those that undermine your efforts to reach long-term goals, as well as those that help move you towards your goals.

Your day is filled with a string of habits.

For example, when the alarm goes off in the morning, do you have to make a conscious decision to brush your teeth, use the bathroom, take a shower, or get dressed? What about looking at your phone?

Probably not.

What about the things you say to yourself when the alarm goes off? Do they make you jump out of bed or hit the snooze button and hide under the covers?

Make no mistake, when it comes to habits, your thoughts — not the time or the place or an emotion or a person or a preceding event — are the real triggers for both action and inaction.

By trigger, I mean the thing that sets a particular habit in motion.

What was the trigger for Tina Fey?

Before you started reading this chapter, you may have answered "the events in Charlottesville" or "the election result" — because it wasn't the one she wanted.

But why did she feel awful? It was what she thought about it and, more specifically, what she was making the outcome mean. That was the real trigger for her binging on sheet cake.

To master your triggers, you first need to become aware of these thoughts.

STOPPING SELF-SABOTAGE

ARE YOU FAMILIAR WITH the analogy about the rider and elephant by Jonathan Haidt?[7] It's about the relationship between the conscious, rational mind and the unconscious or subconscious, emotional mind.

The rider is the conscious mind — where logic, reasoning, and planning take place. It sits atop the more powerful elephant, which is everything else — the

Your ***thoughts*** *are the real*

triggers *for both* ***action***

and ***inaction.***

automatic processes and layers upon layers of unexamined suppositions and experiences — taking place below the level of our awareness.

To stay on any given path, the elephant and rider must be in agreement.

Mastering your triggers, then, is about uncovering both the conscious and subconscious thoughts and beliefs you have, so you give yourself the opportunity to reflect on and reframe them if needed, lest the elephant go on a stampede.

Again, triggers are the thoughts that set your habits in motion.

To create a new habit, to make sustainable, meaningful change, we need to identify the beliefs you have about yourself and your abilities — often the subconscious ones that are hidden from your view but reveal themselves in what you say and what you do — and make sure they are *congruent* with the outcomes you desire.

To do this, we need to take a closer look at the beliefs you have about yourself, both the ones that limit and the ones that lift you.

They're the words you choose to finish a sentence that starts with "I am" and the thoughts about yourself you *actually* believe — not the ones you *want* to believe.

Because those are the ones driving most of your habits and determining the trajectory of your life. You need to uncover them. This is the first step to tapping into the power of your thoughts to generate positive emotions.

Discovery

It was 3:30 a.m., and Diana couldn't sleep. Despite being physically exhausted and emotionally spent after her 12-hour shift, she had been lying awake in bed for the past two hours.

It was May of 2020, and the coronavirus was spreading at an alarming rate through Minneapolis, Minnesota.

Diana, an ER nurse, loved her job, but this pandemic was heart-wrenching. One of her patients had walked in complaining of difficulty breathing the day before and was now on a ventilator. She knew his prognosis wasn't good.

She was worried for her own family, too, because earlier that night, the nurse manager had informed her that because of the staffing shortages, the hospital needed her to cover more shifts, from twice a week to four times a week.

She had never been a good sleeper, and she really needed extra days to recover. Scott, her husband, was a physician at the same public hospital, and they were working opposite 12-hour shifts so the kids wouldn't be home alone. With the schools closed, she had to get up at 7:30 a.m. and take care of them.

If she couldn't get at least five hours of sleep, how was she going to function? Worse, given the stress and sleep deprivation, she knew her immune system would be weaker. What if she came down with Covid herself?

Without sleeping in as an option, she was at a loss. She'd tried melatonin before. It did nothing for her, and sleep aids made her groggy.

"Maybe listening to a podcast can help me fall asleep," she said to herself in desperation. The first episode in the queue happened to be one of mine. The topic was "Recognizing Self-Sabotage." About 10 minutes into the episode, she realized that what others were doing with food, she was doing with sleep.

Seeing a glimmer of hope, she decided this would be a topic for our next coaching session.

With that, she rolled over and finally drifted off to sleep.

Making the Shift

It had been six weeks since Diana had signed up for Joyful Eating Circles, my habit-coaching program for weight loss. She had been working on eating more fruits and vegetables, and we were making steady progress, but she had hesitated to bring up her issues with sleep.

Now she was ready. At our next coaching session, she admitted, "My real issue is sleep. I'm not a good sleeper, never have been."

"My husband has begged me to go see a sleep doctor, but I just didn't believe it would change anything," she continued. "But before I started this program, I didn't think I liked vegetables either," she added. "And now we're averaging 4-5 servings a day. I had really underestimated how important mindset is."

For the rest of the coaching session, we focused on sleep.

I asked what success would look like, and she told me hesitantly, "It would be a dream come true if I could fall asleep within 15 minutes of my head hitting the pillow."

"Have you ever been able to do that?" I asked. I wanted to make sure Diana's sleep problems weren't physiological in nature.

"Come to think of it, yes," Diana said as her forehead smoothed. "About seven years ago, when we were in Bali. My husband was at a conference, and I tagged along. It was glorious. I went to bed around 9 p.m. every night and got up at 6 a.m."

"So, it's possible?" I asked to confirm.

"Yes," Diana replied. Then she smiled. "I just need it to happen on this continent."

New Routines

After Diana described her routines for a typical week, it became clear she didn't have a bedtime routine.

When she couldn't fall asleep, she usually slept in until 10 or 11 a.m. since her husband took the kids to school. Often, she would fall asleep with her daughter around 8:30 p.m. and wake up around 10 p.m.

"When you were in Bali, what do you think helped?" I asked.

When she couldn't think of anything, I offered a few suggestions to help with the brainstorming.

"Did you have a bedtime routine in Bali?" I asked.

"Actually, yes," she answered. "I would brush my teeth, wash my face, take a hot bath, change into my pajamas, and then read a book for 30 minutes before turning out the light."

"Would you be able to do something like that now?" I asked.

"Well, I can definitely do something on the nights I'm not working," she replied.

"And what about waking up at the same time every day? You did that in Bali. Could you do that now?" I continued.

"Yes," she answered.

"Which one feels more doable," I asked, "the bedtime routine or getting up at the same time every day, regardless of when you fall asleep?"

"Well, I can definitely control what time I set the alarm for and get up, so probably that," she answered.

Two weeks later, at our check-in call, she had been able to get up at 7:30 a.m. on all but two of the days. She also noticed that falling asleep wasn't taking as long on the nights after she worked.

"I'm ready to try putting a bedtime routine in place," she volunteered.

"Great! I think you're ready, too. Would this be something you do every night, even nights you're working?" I asked.

"I think it would be better to commit to just the nights I'm not working for now," she replied.

After a bit more fine-tuning, she had a routine that looked very similar to the one in Bali, except instead of reading a book for 30 minutes, she decided some yoga stretches and listening to an audiobook for 30 minutes would be more relaxing.

I reminded her to focus on experimenting and paying attention to what didn't work as well as what did.

Better Results

Six weeks later, her dream came true.

Even though she hadn't left work until 1:30 a.m. — her shift had ended at midnight — she got home and used her bedtime routine to wind down. By the time the automatic timer for the audiobook shut off 30 minutes later, Diana was sound asleep.

These days, Diana considers herself a good sleeper and gets seven to eight hours of sleep on most nights.

And with her sleep routine in place, she noticed she had more energy and more patience. Even her cravings went away.

We continued working together to uncover and identify the self-sabotaging thoughts and behaviors that undermined her efforts, and after another six months, she had the Fundamental Five habits on autopilot.

She now appreciates how much her body responds to the self-care practices she's put in place.

Oh, and she never got Covid.

HOW THE BRAIN WORKS

YOUR BRAIN IS A problem-solving machine. Ask a question, and it's like a search engine looking for an answer.

When Diana asked herself, "Why is sleep such a struggle?" her brain came up with, "Because you've never been a good sleeper."

If your brain recognizes a pattern from the past, it will cue a particular routine that it's used before, a solution that has led to a reward.

Again, the reward doesn't have to be what we normally think of as the carrot. It doesn't have to release happy hormones. It can be simply to avoid pain. If a solution provides both, it will be even more attractive.

That's why, for example, emotional eating is such an easy habit to form. You get a quick dopamine hit from eating, and you get to avoid discomfort.

The discomfort of uncertainty also means our brain prefers quick results. That's why we prefer immediate gratification, even if the reward for delayed gratification is better.

Your brain is ready to tap the brakes at any time. If it perceives a threat, it triggers a stress response — and the release of hormones like cortisol and adrenaline — and your sympathetic nervous system is activated, increasing your heart rate and blood pressure.

And the stress response puts you in survival mode, what you often hear referred to as fight, flight, freeze, or fawn (trying to please to avoid conflict). In this state, there are no resources available for change and growth.

Braking means the actions you take now are not going to align with what you wanted to do when you were in planning mode.

For Diana, just the thought of struggling to fall asleep was enough to trigger stress.

And before we started working together, she would sabotage her sleep efforts with activities that would make falling asleep harder — like falling asleep with her daughter when she put her to bed at 8:30 p.m. This reinforced the belief she had about not being a good sleeper.

This is exactly why awareness of your thoughts is the key to creating change, so you're not driving with one foot on the gas and the other on the brake. By the way, if the elephant is in charge, it's more like the emergency brake. Do you smell the brake pads burning?

When you become aware of your thoughts, you have an opportunity to override the stress response.

You can train your brain to notice and pay attention to different things.

Of course, your self-limiting beliefs may not change overnight. It's a process, and it's easy to forget new insights if you don't take steps to reinforce the new beliefs. This is one reason why journaling can be so helpful. You have an opportunity to capture the insights and refer back to them.

You only need a small crack in the limiting-belief wall where you can insert a wedge. Then, over time, you can give your brain evidence — new instances showing how the old belief doesn't hold true — so you can let go of those limiting beliefs and make room for new ones.

For Diana, the small crack was the time when she was in Bali and was a good sleeper.

Change can be hard, especially after the initial excitement of starting a new habit wanes. But it's important to know and remember that it's not always going to require so much energy and all that conscious, intentional thought.

Remember...

- Becoming aware of your thoughts is key to creating new habits.

- For lasting change, the conscious mind and subconscious mind must be congruent.

- Be mindful of your thoughts, for they are the triggers that set your habits in motion.

In the next chapter, you'll learn how to shift from a state of scarcity to one of abundance, the key to mastering your triggers.

Chapter 4

MASTER YOUR TRIGGERS

WHY IS IT SO hard to make choices that align with your long-term goals?

The answer lies in your biology.

This is why you'll want to focus on the Fundamental Five habits as you begin the process of losing weight for the last time — to make sure you're not in a state of physiological or psychological scarcity.

Remember, any time your brain perceives that your wants and needs are at risk of not being met, the uncertainty triggers a stress response. This is your subconscious brain at work, and it's lightning fast.

Furthermore, your brain cannot tell the difference between a real physical threat and an imagined one. Is a bear threatening to chase you down, or are you just imagining it happening? Brain scans would show the same areas of your brain being activated.[8]

Any time your **brain perceives** *that your wants and needs are* **at risk of not being met,** *the uncertainty triggers a* **stress response.**

Worried about a big presentation you're giving? Your brain lights up just like it would if an actual bear was chasing you.

No wonder you can't fall asleep!

Seriously, if your survival was really at stake, taking a nap would be the last thing you would want to do. So, let's be grateful for that kind of stress response.

The threat response is also based on the underlying assumption that you lack the time and resources needed — or in the case of the presentation, the fear that it's not good enough, something will go wrong, and you won't be able to recover.

So, you ask, "Is there a way to shift from a state of scarcity to one of abundance?"

Yes.

There's a moment of decision where you can make a deliberate intentional choice before that memorized routine kicks in — if you're aware of the thought and take time to ask some questions.

THE POWER OF THE PAUSE

"Between stimulus and response there is a space. In that space is our power to choose our response. In our response lies our growth and our freedom." — Viktor Frankl

TRIGGERS ARE ACTUALLY THE interpretations that drive our emotions, our actions, and, ultimately, our results. These results become the evidence our brain uses to reinforce its mental models for understanding the world.

Your interpretations go through a belief filter.

When it comes to breaking old habits that no longer serve you — like emotional eating, procrastination, not drinking enough water, late-night snacking, skimping on sleep, or avoiding exercise — as well as building new ones for the life you are creating, mastering your triggers is about uncovering self-limiting beliefs and replacing them with self-lifting ones.

This happens in the space between stimulus — your interpretation — and response — the emotion. In other words, when you become aware of a triggering thought, you are going to insert a pause.

HOW TO MAKE THE SHIFT

IT WAS MY FRIEND Cheryl's 50th birthday, and we were celebrating at Maya restaurant in Sonoma. Actually, she had turned 50 two weeks prior, but as the chief product officer of a large software company, she lived in hotels two weeks out of every month, so it wasn't easy finding a time we could meet.

As she perused the menu, she spotted a pasta dish that piqued her interest.

"I would order the Maya Spaghetti, but I can't eat pasta," she said.

"What do you mean you can't eat pasta?" I asked. "You're half Italian. Don't you love pasta?"

"Yes, I do, but I need to lose some weight, so I'm avoiding carbs," she replied.

I knew that Cheryl had used the ketogenic diet before her wedding to lose a significant amount of weight.

"Is it all carbs?" I asked.

"No, I'm giving myself permission to eat fruits and vegetables," she replied.

"What happens when you do eat pasta? How do you feel?" I asked, gathering more information.

"It's like I lose control. Since I only have it on special occasions, I'll keep eating until I'm stuffed, and then I feel miserable. And, of course, I feel guilty because I wasn't supposed to eat it," she sighed. "I need more willpower."

I've known Cheryl for more than 20 years, since our days at Netscape when I hired her as the marketing coordinator for my department. Even then, I could see how much potential she had.

I also knew about her lifelong struggle with weight, and, the bigger concern, her family history of Type 2 diabetes. Her father died of complications from the disease when she was only 16.

"What if the problem isn't pasta, but your thoughts about pasta and the conclusions you're drawing?" I asked. "First, because of the way your brain works, when you tell yourself you can't have it, part of your brain is monitoring to make sure you're not doing it, and you wind up thinking about it more," I explained. "That's why you feel like you need more willpower."

"Second, you're creating an artificial state of scarcity," I continued. "Artificial because clearly, you could get pasta any time. We're not experiencing a pasta famine, right?"

Cheryl smiled as she nodded.

"So, your brain sees this deprivation as a threat, which then triggers a threat response. Basically, it perceives that your wants and needs are at risk of not being met, so then whatever change you're trying to implement is discarded. It's almost impossible to make conscious, intentional decisions when the threat response is triggered," I continued.

I watched as Cheryl absorbed what I was saying. Her head tilted to one side as she pressed her lips together.

"Go ahead. Spit it out," I nudged her with a grin.

"So, I've been making it harder on myself all this time?" she asked, as her brow furrowed. "It can't be that simple."

"Well, yes and no. Yes, you've been making it unnecessarily harder. And no, it's not quite that simple, but it's an important piece of the puzzle. What you're telling yourself creates a state of psychological scarcity, but you may also be doing some things that create a physiological state of scarcity too. Like not getting enough sleep, especially with all the travel you do, which makes losing weight hard. And scarcity of any kind makes it hard to form habits," I responded.

"Anyway, it's your birthday. I say order whatever you want," I said.

"Well, I'll have an extra glass of wine and dessert to celebrate. But I'm still going to skip the pasta," she said.

The next day, Cheryl called me at lunchtime. "So, just to be clear, are you saying I can have pasta and lose weight?" she asked.

"Would it be worth it to you to find out?" I responded.

"Let's do it." she declared.

Two weeks later, we were on a group coaching call, and I presented the diagram of The Learning Cycle or TLC.

With Cheryl's permission, I walked everyone through how to apply it to her situation with pasta.

The Learning Cycle

Situation. *In any given situation, your brain takes in data.*

In this case, we were at a restaurant with various sights and smells, looking at a menu. It was dinner time, and both of us were hungry and getting hungrier by the minute.

Figure 2: The Learning Cycle

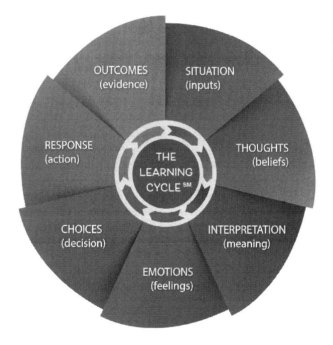

Thoughts. *The data triggers thoughts, including beliefs, facts, and opinions about the situation, and the brain uses these as filters to determine what to focus on and what to ignore. The tricky thing about beliefs and opinions is that we often accept them as facts, no questions asked. You can also think of these*

filters as your brain looking for a familiar mental model to make sense of the current data.

For example, the thoughts Cheryl shared with me included:

- I see a pasta dish that I think I would like.

- I need to lose weight.

- I love pasta.

- Carbs should be avoided for weight loss.

- I need more willpower.

- When I avoided carbs before my wedding, I lost weight.

Can you differentiate the facts from the opinions and beliefs?

If you guessed, "I need to lose weight," is an opinion and then "Carbs should be avoided for weight loss" and "I need more willpower" are beliefs (and to some extent, opinions, too), and the rest are facts, you'd be right.

I'll be talking more about these beliefs and dieting rules in Chapter 6, Free Yourself from Diet Culture.

Interpretation. *This is your perception of reality. The filters are your beliefs. And most of the time, you probably don't question whether the underlying assumptions and resulting interpretations are accurate.*

*The tricky thing about **beliefs** and **opinions** is that we often accept them as **facts**, no questions asked.*

For Cheryl, one of the interpretations or conclusions was, "I can't eat pasta if I want to lose weight." Another one was that "I'll lose control and eat until I'm stuffed."

Emotion. *It's actually your interpretations — and more often than not, what you make it mean about you — that drive your emotions.*

Cheryl expressed feelings of desire for pasta, deprivation when thinking about avoiding it, guilt about eating pasta, fear of losing control, and feeling miserable after overeating.

Can you identify the less obvious limiting belief?

That's right. The statement "I need more willpower" is a limiting belief. Also, I wanted to find out why Cheryl thought she needed to lose weight.

Choices. *In any situation, there are at least two ways you can respond, but usually many more.*

Did you notice there was a lot of all-or-nothing thinking happening here? For example, one binary choice was simply whether or not Cheryl was going to order the pasta dish.

Can you identify what other all-or-nothing thinking was happening?

Take your time.

I'll give you a minute...

Okay, did you pick up on the fear that if she did order the pasta, she would wind up eating it all? And did it occur to you that she could've shared some with me? Or asked for a "to go" box or simply left some on her plate?

Response. *The action or actions you take will be the ones that align best with the thoughts and emotions preceding it/them, and specifically, the actions that align with your self-image — in other words, the beliefs you have about yourself.*

In Cheryl's case, her beliefs and interpretations drove her fears around eating pasta, which aligned with her decision not to order it.

Outcomes. *Based on your response, there will be some kind of outcome, and whether or not you realize it, your brain uses this outcome as evidence that your interpretation was correct.*

The Abundance Principle

Do you make better decisions and choices for your long-term goals when you're in a happy mood, had a good night's sleep, and are feeling confident, or when you're tired, stressed, hungry, and feeling down?

Of course, you make better choices when you're feeling good. We all do.

Why? Because making your choices when you're in a state of abundance is where the magic happens.

"What the heck is a state of abundance?" you ask.

Think about the word "harvest." What does it mean, and what is required for a harvest to occur?

A harvest is when you reap the fruits of your labor.

You plant seeds. You believe you have the time it will take for them to grow, so you nurture them. You give them food and water and plenty of sunshine. Perhaps you even talk to them. You create the conditions to increase the chances of the outcome you desire. The things described here are things *you can control.*

As a result, they thrive.

Of course, this presumes there's not a flood or drought or some other calamity, which *you cannot control.*

A state of abundance is when you believe you have what you need or have access to the resources you need.

Interestingly, when it comes to stress, there are two kinds. One is distress, also known as the threat response and the cause of chronic stress. The other is eustress, also known as the challenge response.

Eustress is the kind of stress response you want to trigger because it means you believe you have what it takes to respond successfully to the situation before you. It's how you grow and get stronger and better.

It's also what leads to flow states or what athletes call being "in the zone." It's how you build resilience.

Other examples?

When you feel gratitude, you're in a state of abundance.

When you feel loved, you're in a state of abundance.

When you see your choices on a continuum, you're in a state of abundance.

When you embrace your moxie, you're in a state of abundance.

When you're playing the long game, you're in a state of abundance.

PRACTICING TLC: THE FOUR-STEP REFRAMING METHOD

BACK TO THE PAUSE...

To master your triggers, you'll be applying The Learning Cycle (TLC) and the Four-Step Reframing Method during the pause.

Here are the steps and a description of how Cheryl used them to reframe her experience with pasta.

Step One: Become aware of your thoughts, especially your inner critic.

You want to focus on the ingrained thought patterns, often subconscious, that no longer serve you.

It's like your commute from work to home. You don't usually have to think about the navigation. But if you want to make a stop on the way home, you've got to be paying attention.

Look for the following phrases:

- "I should" – Judging, good or bad, right or wrong

- "Why can't I" – Your brain is a search engine. It will go searching for an answer to this question.

- "Have to" or "need to" – Judging

- "I can't" – Demotivating

- "What if" – We all have a negativity bias, which means our brains tend to look for worst-case scenarios unless we consciously and intentionally focus our attention on something different.

Cheryl's thoughts were riddled with these phrases: "I need to lose weight," "I can't have pasta," and "I should avoid carbs." If you want to improve your awareness of your thoughts, meditation is a great option.

Step Two: Shine a light on them. Capture your thoughts by writing them down so you can evaluate them like a neutral observer.

Have you ever woken up right in the middle of or after a dream, and for a few minutes, you can remember the dream? But then the memory fades away.

When you uncover ingrained thought patterns, they'll be fleeting, like the dream. Journaling can be an effective way to capture them before you forget them, so you can look at them objectively in the light of day.

Cheryl began to journal about what happened in different situations, separating facts from beliefs, opinions, and interpretations and reframing them.

Step Three: Question the premise.

You've probably heard the expression, "Sunlight is the best disinfectant." Putting your thoughts on a table and being able to examine them in the light of day is very different from letting them bounce around inside your head.

So, imagine putting the thought, belief, interpretation, or conclusion on a table. Objectively evaluate it, and ask, "Is this true?"

Seriously, I want you to challenge the premise. Can you think of an instance when it hasn't been true? And what does that mean for you?

Then, if it *is* true, ask yourself if it's helpful. Or, are you operating from a place of fear — fear of the process, fear of the outcome, or fear of loss?

Remember: Fear is one of the negative emotions triggered when our brains interpret a situation as one where our wants and needs are NOT going to be met.

Next, is it kind?

Last, is it necessary?

For Cheryl, the thought, "I should avoid carbs," meant she couldn't eat one of her favorite foods. This was unsustainable and the first interpretation we examined.

Step Four: Reframe your interpretation where needed.

Here's where you want to apply the Abundance Principle.

Whatever the interpretation of the situation is, the easiest way to reframe it so you experience the situation from a state of abundance is to widen the lens so you can see it from a different perspective. And then utilize a very important skill called perceptual positioning.

In human interactions, there are four positions of perception. The first is from your own perspective. The second is from the other person's or people's perspective. The third is from a neutral observer's position. And the fourth is from a position of observing the observer.

Usually, when we talk about empathy, we're referring to emotional empathy, the ability to feel what someone else is feeling.

With perceptual positioning, we're relying on cognitive empathy. This is about understanding what someone else is thinking, how they would feel, and how they would respond as a result. The key difference between emotional empathy and cognitive empathy is that with the latter, you're able to maintain your objectivity.

This is one of the biggest reasons why you want to work with a coach. I can more easily see your situation as a neutral observer. Think of it as a bottle with a label. As a coach, I'm on the outside, whereas you're trying to read the label from inside the bottle.

When reframing, you want to look at a given situation from these different positions. It will help you build self-awareness, better your understanding and empathy skills, and discover new insights into any situation or relationship.

An effective way to shift into these different positions is to ask the following questions:

What am I making this mean about me?

What if the opposite is true?

What else could it mean?

What information am I missing?

Cheryl learned how to notice her urges and name the emotions she was feeling, and journaling definitely helped.

She also learned how powerful her thoughts are, how to recognize triggers of scarcity, how to insert a pause and create the space to question the accuracy of her interpretations, and how to shift her perspective to reframe them.

Instead of abstaining from pasta, Cheryl gave herself permission to eat it as long as she was hungry.

We talked about the Hunger Scale (see Figure 3), the benefits of eating when she's hungry (at -4) and stopping when she's comfortably full (at +4), learning how to sense the edges of her hunger and fullness, without guilt or restriction, and eating more mindfully and joyfully.

Figure 3: Hunger Scale

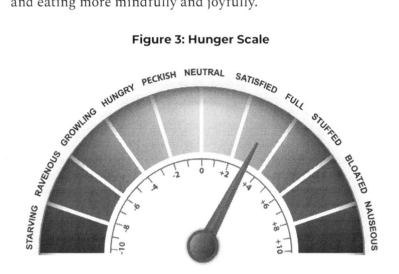

In other words, instead of telling herself, "You can't have it," and creating resistance to an invisible external force, she asked herself, "Have you had enough?" and gave the power and control back to herself.

Every time Cheryl became aware of a triggering thought, she used the Practice TLC worksheet (included in the Bonus) to examine the thought.

It worked. As a matter of fact, during our annual holiday shopping excursion, she said to me, "I have a bone to pick with you. I lost so much weight during the last eight months that all of my pants are too loose. I have to add new pants to my list of things to buy."

"Oh, darn," I replied with a grin.

Then she added, "Who knew I could eat pasta three times a week and still lose weight?"

By the way, she wound up losing 28 pounds over the course of 10 months. And she donated all the clothes that no longer fit.

MAKING HABITS STICK

LEARNING HOW TO MASTER your triggers isn't just to stop thought and behavior patterns that don't serve you. It's also how you make healthy habits stick.

When you take action because you feel good about the process and the result, you're triggering states of abundance. That's when behaviors become easy and sustainable. (More of this in Chapter 7.)

Remember...

- The key to mastering your triggers is examining your thoughts.

- Human behavior doesn't just happen. It's motivated by an anticipated payoff.

- When you become aware of a triggering thought, use the power of the pause to reflect and reframe.

In the next chapter, we'll be identifying the specific habits and practices of Joyful Eating. This is about connecting the dots from where you are now to where you're going, so you can start enjoying the benefits of being the healthy eater you're becoming.

Chapter 5

REDISCOVER JOYFUL EATING

"What you get by achieving your goals is not as important as what you become by achieving your goals." — Henry David Thoreau

AS YOU WAVE GOODBYE to the weight loss struggle bus, welcome to the home of Joyful Eating. *Mi casa es tu casa.*

Here you'll learn about the habits and practices of the Joyful Eating Framework™. And you'll be taking care of your body and giving it what it needs. You'll also be creating a healthy relationship with food, forming a positive body image, and cultivating healthy relationships with friends and family.

WHAT IS JOYFUL EATING?

HAVE YOU EVER WATCHED a baby nursing? I was six years old when my sister, Angela, was born, and I can still remember watching with fascination as my mom breastfed her.

As a baby, my sister had a distinctive cry when she was getting hungry, which, of course, immediately stopped as soon as she latched on to my mother's breast and started sucking the warm milk from it.

There was focus — a baby's version of mindful eating. Mom requested, "No distractions, please."

Sometimes my sister would hold my mom's finger — comforting, no doubt.

Safe and warm in my mom's loving arms, my sister trusted her needs would be met.

And when she was comfortably full, she was done. Full stop. Content and satisfied. No external rules to abide by and certainly no feelings of guilt.

This was joyful eating.

So simple.

Chances are, when you were a baby, you had a similar experience. And when you look at photos from your past, you probably have birthday celebrations as a child with cake and ice cream and a big smile on your face.

You were still enjoying the moments, surrounded by friends and family.

This is why, when I refer to joyful eating, I use the word "rediscover."

THE FOUR PILLARS

ALLOW ME TO INTRODUCE you to the Joyful Eating Framework, its four pillars — love, nourishment, trust, and gratitude — and the habits and practices of a healthy eater.

Figure 4: Joyful Eating Framework™

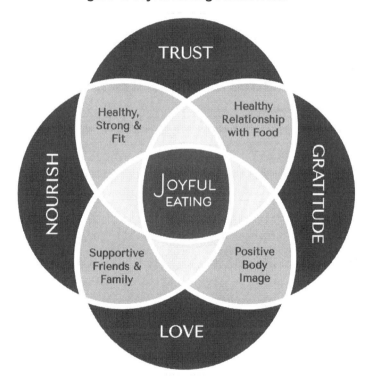

Speaking of mi casa, I want you to imagine you're looking at the blueprint for not just a house but a home.

What would you expect to find?

Love, of course! The first pillar of Joyful Eating is love. In your mind's eye, picture a bedroom.

With love, there's acceptance instead of self-loathing. There are healthy boundaries, and we approach life's struggles with compassion.

Instead of disparaging your body, you cherish your life, your body, your health, and your talents.

Imagine yourself as a child, that perfect little being, and think about what you would be doing to take care of that little person.

"When you love someone, you love the person as they are, and not as you'd like them to be." — Leo Tolstoy

First and foremost, you would be coming from a place of love.

And unconditional love is about accepting the person — namely, you — just the way you are. You need to know that your intrinsic value — your worth — isn't about the number on the scale or how you look, what you do, or how much you've accomplished.

You are precious and worth taking care of.

You deserve to feel better.

You are already enough.

As you gain clarity on your wants and needs and preferences — that is, your boundaries — you'll figure out what foods you truly like to eat, how much sleep you need to be well-rested, what kinds of movement feel good....

This list goes on.

Instead of listening to the inner critic when your efforts hit the predictable bumps, roadblocks, and detours, you'll

With **love,** there's

acceptance instead

of **self-loathing.**

practice kindness and compassion with yourself as much as you do with others. You'll realize the health and happiness journey isn't about what you achieve but who you become as you achieve your goals, one by one.

The second pillar is nourishment. Think of it as the kitchen.

This is where you'll be nourishing your mind, body, and soul. Using Maslow's hierarchy[9] of needs to inform the process, you'll start with the Fundamental Five Habits. Beyond those, you'll be cultivating relationships, approaching life with curiosity and learning, and building resilience.

When you think of nourishment, think about habits and practices that move you from abusing to caring for your brain and body.

You'll start paying attention to what you can control, like how you nourish your body and how you take care of your mental and emotional health.

Now, instead of worrying about the number of calories, you focus on what's in the food you're eating. Are you getting enough vitamins and minerals? Are you getting enough fiber? Enough protein? Enough fat? Enough water?

You'll focus on things like getting enough sleep and moving your body to keep it strong, fit, and flexible.

You'll process your emotions, so instead of simply coping as best you can with difficult situations, you'll be able to respond effectively and appropriately.

And you'll spend your time with friends and family, one of the keys to longevity and happiness.[10]

The third pillar is trust. Think of it like the floor or foundation.

Trusting your body is about interoception and, more specifically, interoceptive fidelity, which consists of awareness, attunement, and alignment.

Interoception is known as our eighth sense. It's how your brain becomes aware of what's going on inside your body.

Exteroception is the senses focused on how you take in the outside world — what you see, hear, smell, taste, and touch.

Proprioception and vestibular are your sixth and seventh senses. The former is how you perceive the location, movement, and action of different parts of your body. And the latter is how you maintain your balance, how you know the orientation of your head and body and your awareness of movement.

With interoceptive awareness, we become aware of the different sensations in our bodies. These sensations include hunger, thirst, fullness, pain, heat, cold, and fatigue at a fine-tuned level. For example, do you notice when you're somewhat hungry, or do you ignore the signals until you're starving?

With interoceptive attunement, you're able to accurately interpret what the signals mean. Is the headache you're experiencing due to dehydration, tension from stress, or a fever?

And with interoceptive alignment, you're listening to what your body is telling you by responding appropriately.

When you're tired, do you rest, or do you keep pushing until you get sick?

Interoceptive fidelity is about trusting yourself and your body.

And when you trust your body, instead of ignoring its signals, you honor them.

You learn how to listen to it, become aware of the sensations, and understand what they are telling you.

Are you hungry? How hungry are you?

Are you eating because you're physically hungry?

Are you full? Are you satisfied? Have you had enough?

And because your emotions have corresponding physical sensations in the body, you learn to pay attention to these too. See Figure 5.[11]

Because to live life to the fullest, you want to feel all your feelings — the full spectrum. Knowing that, if you avoid the negative ones, inevitably, you'll wind up shortening the spectrum on the positive ones too.

Yes, you'll want the highs to be higher, even if the lows are lower, because you're here for it all.

Figure 5: Bodily Sensation Maps of Emotions

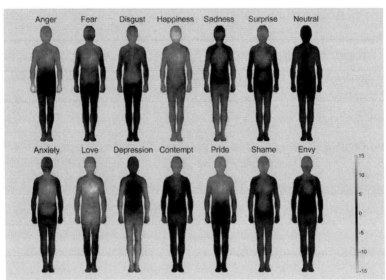

It's not about numbing or avoiding your feelings with food and alcohol. Instead, you've learned to sit with the emotions, let them permeate through you, trust yourself to be able to handle them, and ask for help when needed.

Most of all, you honor them.

And as you become more attuned to what these signals from your body actually mean, you'll be able to align your actions to meet your needs.

In other words, when you're tired, you'll rest. When you're hungry, you'll eat. When you're thirsty, you'll drink. When you're angry, you'll insert a pause. When you're grieving, you'll sit with the emotion.

The fourth pillar is gratitude. Think of it as the roof.

When were you ever not grateful to have a roof over your head?

With gratitude, you'll be using The Learning Cycle to reflect, reframe, and then reclaim your power. For example, instead of punishing your body with exercise to shrink it, you'll be appreciating all your body does to help you accomplish what you want.

Joyful Eating is a self-care framework to help you create the optimal conditions for a happy and healthy life. It's about falling in love with the process, so instead of chasing the outcomes associated with intentional weight loss, the outcomes are simply the eventual by-products.

My hope for you is that through this framework, you'll be showing up as the best version of yourself, growing, learning, connecting, and creating the life you want.

MAKING PEACE WITH FOOD

BETH WAS FEELING ON top of the world.

After receiving a standing ovation for her keynote address, she mingled with her admirers at the post-event cocktail party.

"Great presentation, Beth!"

"You really knocked that one out of the park!"

It was October 2016. Beth, the senior vice president of business development at a major investment bank, was attending a prestigious financial technology conference where investors went to identify and woo the founders of seed-stage startups for their companies to take public.

At the post-event cocktail party, she spotted someone she wanted to talk with — Peter, the CFO of the startup her company had been courting for the past six months.

Just at that moment, she walked past the hors d'oeuvres table, where she spotted a platter with her favorite cheese and olive oil crackers.

Uh oh!

She felt herself turn toward the tray and start reaching for one. And then she stopped herself. She knew if she had one, it would be like breaking the dam. After battling with her weight for years, her cravings for simple cheese and crackers had gotten worse and worse. It was her kryptonite.

"This is not part of the diet," she reminded herself.

She was 60 pounds overweight, and she was always thinking about this in the back of her mind. She had struggled with her weight since the birth of her second son, and it had led to the knee problems she now was having.

"Use your willpower," she said, trying to refocus.

By the time she looked back up, Peter was leaving with one of her company's competitors.

"Damn it," she said to herself.

Suppressing a moan, she reached for a plate and proceeded to fill it with whatever looked good as her frustration and anger with herself mounted.

The first bite of the cheese and crackers were a welcome distraction and temporary relief as the salt hit her taste buds.

But when the plate was empty, her frustration and anger were still there, with the added burden of guilt for going off her diet.

That night, in bed, she thought about how her cravings had ruined what should've been a moment of victory that she could've been savoring now. They may have cost her company a lucrative client.

"You have to stop these cravings once and for all," she told herself.

She'd been using one of the weight-loss programs some of her friends had found success with, but it wasn't working for her.

She confided in Howard, her husband and biggest supporter, and he suggested she talk to me at the health club to see if I could help her or recommend someone for her to work with. They'd both been members of my health club for a few months, and we were on very friendly terms.

When Beth found out I was not just the owner of the club but also a nutrition and health coach, she met with me that same afternoon.

We started by discussing her weight loss goals and her past efforts.

"Have you tried to lose weight by avoiding carbs? I asked.

"Yes," she replied. "But my issue is cheese and crackers. When I see them, it's like 98 percent of my attention goes to them. I can't focus on anything else."

I explained that when you try not to think of something, one part of your mind follows the instruction while another part continuously checks in to make sure the thought is not coming up — bringing it to mind.

"In an ideal world, what would you like to happen when you see cheese and crackers? I asked.

"I would love to be able to take it or leave it," she replied.

"Got it. I have some exercises I think will help with that. My favorite is the one I call Red Light, Green Light, and it's helped a lot of my clients with triggering foods. Would you like to try it?" I asked.

"Sure," she said, "I'm game."

Red Light, Green Light

I instructed Beth to create three columns on a piece of paper and label the top of each with a different label: "red light," "yellow light," and "green light."

In the red-light column, I asked her to list all the foods she could think of that triggered her when she saw them. Under the green-light column, I asked her to list the foods that weren't an issue at all. And in the yellow-light column, I asked her to list the foods that were only issues under certain circumstances.

Turns out for Beth, the red-light foods tended to be salty and crunchy, like cheese and crackers or chips and salsa. She didn't have a big sweet tooth.

A few days later, on a quiet Saturday afternoon, Beth sat down with a box of her favorite crackers and a block of gouda cheese.

She felt her pulse quicken.

"It's just cheese and crackers," she told herself as she felt a wave of anxiety.

Then she took a deep breath, then another, and she gave herself permission to eat as many as she wanted. She opened the box of crackers and took out 10 crackers. Then, she sliced 10 pieces of cheese and carefully placed one on each cracker.

Usually, she ate an entire cracker in one mouthful. I had asked her to eat them mindfully.

"This'll be interesting," she thought.

As she took the first bite, she told herself to eat slowly and pay attention to the taste and texture, the sound of the crunch as she chewed, and the richness of the cheese as it softened on her tongue.

"So good," she thought.

It was hard to chew slowly.

By the fourth cracker, she noticed she was really thirsty and poured herself a glass of sparkling wine from the refrigerator.

As she started eating the fifth cracker, she thought back to the first time she met Howard, at a friend's birthday party, over a plate of cheese and crackers.

She had forgotten about this detail. No wonder she liked them so much.

THOUGHTS ARE HABITS TOO

By the seventh cracker, she started thinking about other foods and what she had in her refrigerator that she could cook for dinner.

Wait... what?!

"How is it I'm thinking about other food?" Beth asked herself. There were still three crackers left on the plate.

Freedom Around Food

At her next coaching session, I asked Beth if she had had a chance to try the exercise.

She nodded.

"How did it go?" I asked.

"I'm still not sure I believe it, but I didn't wind up eating the whole plate."

"So, this exercise helped with the cravings?" I asked.

"Absolutely," Beth said, nodding and smiling.

Of course, her weight-loss struggle wasn't just about cheese and crackers.

There were other red-light foods on her list and other things she was doing that undermined her weight-loss efforts. For instance, she wasn't eating enough, which was slowing down her metabolism, and she wasn't getting enough sleep, which messed with her entire system. She also used emotional eating as her go-to coping method to deal with stress.

During the coaching session, I shared the Fundamental Five self-care habits as a starting point, a way to lay the foundation for all her efforts, and she decided to prioritize getting seven to nine hours of sleep and eating five servings of fruits and vegetables a day.

Each week, we checked in on the self-care habits she was forming.

And each week, she tackled one of the foods on the list under the red-light column.

We worked on identifying and reframing the thought patterns and beliefs that undermined her efforts.

We shifted thoughts like, "I can't eat carbs if I want to lose weight," by asking if this rule was universally true and by challenging the premise. Then we shifted the control from external — the outside force dictating what you can and can't do — to internal by reframing it to "I am choosing to eat this food because it tastes good and I enjoy eating it."

In addition, we also identified rules from her childhood, like, "You have to clean your plate."

Just three months later, at the company holiday party, Beth ate half a plate of cheese and crackers and threw the other half away, not because she felt guilty, but because she had had enough.

Her journey to making peace with food was well underway, and as she mastered her thought triggers, her cravings subsided.

First Things First

Now that you have all the pieces of the puzzle, the concepts, you need to start putting them into place one at a time. You'll want to start with the Fundamental Five.

Remember...

"Knowing is not enough; we must apply.
Willing is not enough; we must do." — Johann von Goethe

As you work on each of the Fundamental Five self-care habits, think about what role the practices within love, nourishment, trust, and gratitude play in forming them.

Again, the Fundamental Five are:

* 7-9 hours of 😴 sleep

* 1/2 your body weight in ounces of 💧 water

* 5 servings of 🥦🍊 veggies and fruit

* Eat until you're comfortably full 😊

* 30 minutes of mindful 🤸🏋️ movement

THE ROADMAP

TO HELP YOU DETERMINE what areas require the most focus, review the statements below and rate yourself on a scale of 1 to 10, where 1 is "needs work" and 10 is "mastery."

Note: Each one of the statements addresses a specific practice in Joyful Eating. Please keep in mind that each rating is merely an indicator, similar to the check engine light on your car's dashboard.

The Statements

	STATEMENT	RATING	PILLAR	PRACTICE
1.	I believe I am worth taking care of and deserve to feel good.		Love	Acceptance
2.	I know my own wants, needs, and preferences.		Love	Boundaries
3.	When I'm feeling down, I try to approach my feelings with curiosity and openness.		Love	Compassion
4.	I make choices about eating, sleeping, and exercise that create the optimal conditions for physical health.		Nourish	Fundamental Five
5.	I feel excited about taking on new challenges and trying and learning new things.		Nourish	Curiosity
6.	I have routines and activities to help me stay in touch with friends and family, as well as cultivate new relationships.		Nourish	Connection
7.	I'm able to match my emotions with the sensations in my body.		Trust	Awareness

	STATEMENT	RATING	PILLAR	PRACTICE
8.	I'm able to sense the edges of my hunger and fullness.		Trust	Attunement
9.	When I feel tired, I prioritize sleep. I also notice that my body feels rested and more alert after sleeping eight hours, and this makes me more likely to get eight hours of sleep again.		Trust	Alignment
10.	I'm aware of the thoughts and beliefs about thinness that make me feel inferior and lead me to look for a weight loss solution that promises fast, dramatic results.		Gratitude	Reflection
11.	I appreciate that the number on the scale is just one indicator of my overall physical health and a limited one at that. It cannot measure my talents, inner beauty, strength, courage, tenacity, potential, or capacity to love.		Gratitude	Reframing
12.	I'm not afraid of the judgment or criticism of others.		Gratitude	Reclaiming

Your Answers

Find one of each: a red, yellow, and green pen or highlighter.

Now, for each question where you indicated a number between 1 and 5, circle or highlight your answer in red. If the number is between 6 and 8, circle in yellow. If the number is between 9 and 10, circle in green.

Figure 6: Joyful Eating Roadmap

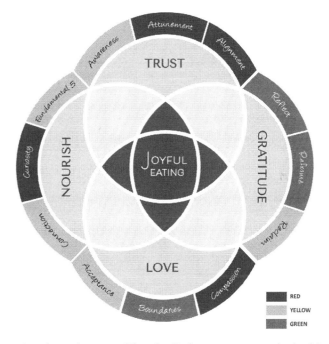

Again, the colors are like the lights on your car's dashboard, letting you know what you may want to check on. The answers circled in green are your areas of strength. Those in yellow need some attention, and those in red require some tender loving care.

THE NEXT BIG STEP

CONGRATULATIONS! YOU'VE COMPLETED A big step in the process. You now have a good visual you can use to map out what Joyful Eating practices you'll want to focus on in the coming weeks and months.

Remember...

- You've experienced joyful eating before. You know how to do it. This is simply the process of rediscovery.

- Focus on creating the optimal conditions for a happy and healthy life. Let the outcomes be the eventual by-products.

- To go from where you are now to where you want to go, start with one of the Fundamental Five Habits.

Now before you go taking a deep dive into one of the habits or practices, there's something else you need to do first. You need to let go.

You need to let go of diet culture beliefs because the underlying beliefs of Joyful Eating are in direct conflict with them.

> *"You can never cross the ocean until you have the courage to lose sight of the shore." — Christopher Columbus*

And the best part? By letting go, you're free to embrace "New & Improved" core beliefs that better serve you.

Ready? We're going to do this in the next chapter.

Chapter 6

FREE YOURSELF FROM DIET CULTURE

"There are these two young fish swimming along and they happen to meet an older fish swimming the other way, who nods at them and says 'Morning, boys. How's the water?' And the two young fish swim on for a bit, and then eventually one of them looks over at the other and goes 'What the hell is water?'" — David Foster Wallace

DIET CULTURE IS EVERYWHERE in the United States. We're literally swimming in it, so it's no wonder we don't question the underlying belief system.

What do I mean?

Well, first, let's take a moment to define culture. Simply put, it's a way of life. It's reflected in the language, values, norms, and beliefs of a particular group, organization, or society.

Figure 7: The Language of Diet Culture

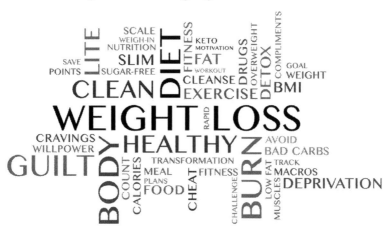

In diet culture, values like appearance and attractiveness, both aspects of outer beauty, take priority over and above everything else — including physical health, mental health, emotional well-being, talent, courage, strength, intelligence, character, wisdom, kindness, and the capacity to love.

And diet culture norms include:

- Chronic dieting for intentional weight loss

- Preoccupation with food

- Restricting certain foods

- Feelings of deprivation and then guilt after eating

- Weekly weigh-ins

- Dreading the need to go up a size in clothing

- The comparison game (where you compare your body with the bodies of others when you walk into a room and decide if yours is more or less attractive)

- A need for external validation (like compliments on weight loss and attractiveness)

- The judgment of others (usually unsolicited comments like "you need to lose weight")

THE UNDERLYING BELIEFS

IF YOU'RE COMPARING YOURSELF to photoshopped images on magazine covers or filtered photos on social media, it's not surprising if you're unhappy with the way you look.

It's also no wonder you avoid the camera, dread wearing shorts and bathing suits, and wind up sitting on the sidelines of life, telling yourself, "When I lose the weight, then I'll be happy."

If you buy into what diet culture is promoting, no matter what you look like or how much you weigh, you're likely to still feel like you're less than and never enough — not thin enough, not pretty enough, not toned enough.

Or maybe you wish you still weighed what you did a year ago, or five years ago, or back in college.

These feelings of "not enough" stem from the following beliefs, which are the basis of diet culture:

- Thinness is an outward reflection of health, especially for women.

- Being thin, toned, and young is considered more attractive for women.

- Eating healthier food makes you more disciplined and, therefore, a better person.

- Those who are thin and young are of higher value in society.

And, at the same time, diet culture conveys messages like:

- Having extra fat on your body means you lack self-control or love food too much, are less healthy than those who are thin, are less attractive or are unattractive, and should be ashamed about the size and shape of your body.

- If you're not attractive enough, you could wind up unmarried — an old maid, alone and childless.

In the end, it's easy to see how the size and shape of your body can be conflated with your sense of self-worth.

DEFUNDING THE FOOD POLICE

IF YOU WANT TO become a healthy eater, if you want to experience joyful eating, you'll need to let go of the beliefs and rules that no longer serve you.

If you want to experience *joyful eating,* you'll need to **let go** of the beliefs and rules that **no longer serve you.**

Otherwise, it's like trying to drive with the parking brake on, swimming with a weight attached to your ankle, or sailing with your anchor down. Pick the metaphor that will help you remember.

Here are some additional statements from diet culture (and perhaps rules you grew up with) that you may have accepted as true and internalized:

*You should avoid "bad" carbs and fat
if you want to lose weight.*

You should clean your plate.

*You can have some ice cream as a
reward after you finish your homework.*

You'll be healthier when you lose weight.

Going on a diet is how you lose weight.

You need to exercise in order to lose weight.

Fitness challenges can help you lose 20 pounds in 30 days.

You need to have a flat tummy to rock a bikini.

You won't be lovable if you're fat.

Just lose the weight first. Then figure out how to maintain it.

If you still find yourself lured by the promises of diets, consider this: If diet and weight-loss programs actually helped people lose weight for good, would that industry be worth $175 billion in the US?[12]

Best case: These programs are simply ineffective. Worse case: Their ineffectiveness is how they ensure they have repeat customers.

UNWITTING CONSPIRATORS

TO MAKE MATTERS WORSE, most physicians use your body mass index or BMI as a key metric in determining whether your weight is in what is considered the normal or healthy range.

Unfortunately, BMI measurements don't take your body composition into account. As a result, two individuals who are the same height can have the same BMI but very different amounts of body fat and lean body mass.

And the BMI ranges for determining underweight, normal, overweight, and obese are based primarily on data collected from non-Hispanic white populations. This means it doesn't take into account a person's body shape, gender, age, race, or ethnicity.

In other words, there's a built-in bias. Someone who is big-boned and very muscular could wind up in the overweight range even though they actually have less fat and a healthier body composition than a smaller-boned, less muscular counterpart.

No doubt your doctor is concerned about your physical health. But at what expense?

Seriously, have you ever postponed a doctor's visit because you didn't want to step on the scale and hear some version of "you need to lose weight" from a well-intentioned physician?

If avoiding the doctor leads to a delay in the diagnosis and treatment of a serious disease, the outcomes could be far worse than a few extra pounds.

Also, by focusing only on having patients lose weight for physical health and to manage conditions like high blood pressure and type 2 diabetes, physicians often discount or altogether ignore the resulting negative effects on their patients' mental and emotional health — the stress from dieting and the frustration of weight cycling.

If your goal is to lose weight and keep it off, freeing yourself of diet culture will go a long way in helping you ignore the quick-fix solutions and lean into the self-care habits that make lasting weight loss easy and inevitable. To do this, you need to become aware of when you're under diet culture's influence so you can take appropriate action.

RECOGNIZING DIET CULTURE

NANCY LOVED HER NEW baby with all her heart.

At eight weeks old, Teddy had beautiful, twinkling eyes, chubby cheeks, and dimples where his elbows and knees were.

When she looked over at him lying in his playpen, napping peacefully, she thought he was perfect.

Sitting on the living-room sofa looking at the photos her husband, Mike, had taken of her playing with Teddy one evening, she cringed. She hated the way she looked in the photos.

"I have to lose this baby weight and get rid of my double chin," she chided herself as she touched her neck.

"Can't you just enjoy the moment?" Mike said.

There was a long pause as tears welled up in Nancy's eyes, and her throat tightened. She and Mike were both sleep-deprived and short-tempered. Between the raging hormones and lack of sleep, Nancy couldn't think straight.

"What's wrong with me?" she asked herself and felt a wave of sadness and loneliness wash over her.

That afternoon, she attended an online nutrition seminar, hoping to glean some new tips on weight loss. I happened to be the guest expert, and after hearing how I helped clients achieve their weight-loss goals by focusing on habits, she decided to hire me as her coach.

We scheduled her initial consultation for the following Monday.

I began by asking her about her background and what she was hoping to get out of the program.

Nancy had gained 30 pounds during her pregnancy. Since giving birth, she had already lost 20 pounds, but her progress had slowed. "I really want to get back to my pre-baby weight," she said. She told me about her job as an assistant professor at a top-tier medical school, her experience as a college athlete in track, and the birth of her son just eight weeks prior.

"What prompted you to reach out to me now rather than, say, a month ago?" I asked.

Nancy then shared what had happened a few days earlier with the photos of herself and her baby. "I see Teddy years from now, showing these photos to a girlfriend and feeling embarrassed," she said, as her voice trailed off.

"Who's embarrassed?" I asked.

"Teddy. Because of how I look. I'm afraid he'll be ashamed of me," she said.

"So you're afraid of what he'll think," I reflected back. "What else are you thinking when you look at the pictures?"

"Well," she said. "In the past month, I've only lost five pounds. So, I have ten more to go. And I really want to get there before my parents visit later this summer because I really want to avoid getting comments from my mom about my weight.

"I come from a family of high achievers," she explained. "Both my parents are physicians, and when I'm with them, I know I'm constantly being judged. I don't like it, although I have to admit it feels great when I get compliments."

And then she sighed. "I wish I didn't care so much about what people think of me."

I nodded. "Including your parents?" I asked.

"Yes. Of course, I want them to be proud of me — what kid doesn't? But it's like nothing short of perfection is acceptable. When I was in high school, after a track meet, unless I came in first place, my parents would barely look at me and wouldn't really say anything."

When Nancy talked about how she had "only lost five pounds," I could hear the disappointment in her voice. When I noted how hard she was being on herself, she insisted that this was how she had gotten to where she was.

And when I asked if she would be happy when she lost the ten pounds, she shook her head and replied, "No, I always worry about gaining it back."

As I listened to Nancy, I heard the language of diet culture peppered throughout her answers.

I shared my observations with her and then walked her through The Learning Cycle and the four-step method for reframing.

Here's a partial list of the thoughts I identified.

- Teddy will be ashamed of the way his mom looks.

- In the past month, I've only lost five pounds.

- I think I look better when I'm thinner.

- I really want to avoid getting comments from my mom about my weight.

- Nothing short of perfection is acceptable.

- I know I'm constantly being judged.

- I'll probably be worried about gaining it back.

For her homework, I asked her to take some time with each statement and see if she could distinguish among those that were facts, opinions, beliefs, and interpretations and then determine what she was making them mean about herself.

I reminded her that opinions are often stated to sound like facts and beliefs and are accepted as true — as if they are facts. Her task was to challenge the premise of each statement and see which ones stood up to scrutiny.

FINDING ACCEPTANCE AND INNER PEACE

NANCY AND I MET again the following week. "Did you get a chance to do the homework?" I asked.

"Yes, and it was really helpful to be able to look at them on paper, to look at them objectively," she replied.

"What did you figure out?" I asked.

"Well, the whole thing with Teddy being embarrassed is from my fears. He obviously doesn't feel that way now, and I have no idea how he'll feel when he's older," Nancy said with relief.

"I love how the exercise was so simple. I looked at the statement, 'Teddy will be embarrassed,' and I asked myself, 'Is this true?' Of course, the answer is no. I was feeling all this shame for something that hasn't even happened yet," she said.

Nancy also figured out that the judgments of other people about her weight — both compliments and criticisms — were just opinions. But she couldn't shake the need for her parents' approval.

I explained that when she seeks external validation — like the approval of her parents — she is basing how she feels on what someone else thinks, and believing she's only good enough if she hears it from someone else, if someone else judges her to be worthy.

Relying on external validation means you're making your happiness dependent on something external to you, over which you have no control.

And if the validation is about something you've achieved, remember your worth is not attached to what you accomplish.

Love is about who you are. Approval is about what you do.

"I'm getting a recording of this, right?" she asked. "This approval thing is gonna take some work."

I nodded and smiled. "Yes, I'll send you the link after our session."

TAKE BACK YOUR POWER

NOW IT'S YOUR TURN. What thoughts do you have — rules about eating, beliefs about beauty standards and your worth — that have gone unexamined?

For some examples, we'll go back to one of the underpinning beliefs of diet culture.

Thinness is an outward reflection of health.

Now that you see this statement in black and white, what do you think? Is it true?

Consider this: One of the symptoms of cancer is unexplained weight loss.

So, what if someone is battling cancer? Or what if someone is grieving the loss of a loved one and has no appetite? Or they're going through a particularly stressful time? Suffering from depression?

What about this one? *Being thin and toned is universally more attractive.*

Can you think of an example that contradicts the assertion?

When you see or hear the reflections of **diet culture,** they only have **power** to affect how you feel about yourself if you **believe** them to be **true.**

What about Marilyn Monroe? Jennifer Lopez? Beyonce Knowles?

Next: *Those who are thin are of higher value and status in society.*

What about Oprah Winfrey?

When you see or hear the reflections of diet culture, they only have power to affect how you feel about yourself if you believe them to be true.

Each and every time you become aware of a belief from diet culture that weighs you down and leaves you feeling less than enough, practice TLC using the Four-Step Reframing Method from Chapter 4. Those negative beliefs will lose their hold on you.

If the thought ultimately equates or conflates your worth with the size and shape of your body, challenge the premise and reframe it.

Eventually, as you uncover these thoughts you've heard, the ones that were unquestioned and internalized, you'll be able to let go of them one by one.

Practice TLC using the worksheets in the companion workbook, which you can download at ThoughtsAreHabitsToo. com/Bonus.

PRACTICING SELF-COMPASSION

"NOW, WHAT ABOUT CRITICISM?" I asked. "If your mom was here right now and said, 'You need to lose weight,' would it bother you?"

"Definitely," Nancy answered.

"Okay, when something's triggering like this, there's another question you need to ask besides, 'Is it true?' and that is, 'What am I making it mean about me?'

"That I'm... oh, I get it! That I'm not enough just the way I am," she said. "But I know my mom loves me," she continued, "and she wants what's best for me."

"And..." I prodded.

"And I'm looking for approval from her about my appearance, which is important, but in the grand scheme of things, not that important. If she believes that losing weight will help me get what I want in life, I can see why she would bring it up. But that doesn't make it right."

I nodded in agreement.

"Wow, I feel a lot better. It really helps to see all of this from a broader context," she smiled and then continued, "But I still think I need to lose weight."

"In other words, you agree with your mom. Do you think that's why it bothers you? Like there's a wound already there, and her comment is rubbing salt in it," I asked.

"Yes," she answered.

"Well, let me ask you this. Would you say it that way to your best friend? Or would you find a kinder, more compassionate way to say it because you want to encourage them to take better care of themselves?"

"Oh, I see. That's what you meant when you said I was being hard on myself," she remarked.

"It's like the T-shirt that says, 'The beatings will continue until morale improves,'" I said. "That's really not the best way to motivate someone. As a matter of fact, when you think about your favorite teachers or managers or mentors, why are they your favorites? How did they make you feel about yourself?

"And please remember, this is all a process," I continued. "We're talking about learning how to be your own best friend. The last thing I would want you to do is start judging yourself on how you're doing this."

Nancy grinned. "I'll try to remember that."

DEBUNKING THE EXERCISE MYTH

"SO, BACK TO WHY you hired me... want to create some new self-care habits and see what happens?"

"Yes," she answered.

I reviewed the Fundamental Five Habits with her and then asked, "Which one would you like to focus on first?"

"Exercise. I'm so flabby," she said while poking her stomach. "But I also want to work on eating more fruits and vegetables. And I could really use more sleep."

I explained that the goal was to build all five habits, and she would eventually get there, but we were going to focus on just one habit at a time. It was important to avoid overwhelm and to give her brain evidence that the process was working.

After some additional discussion, Nancy decided that movement was her highest priority, so to start, we set a goal of two 30-minute workouts per week.

At the beginning of our coaching session, Nancy lamented, "I'm so annoyed with myself that I only managed to get in two workouts."

"I'm confused. Why are you frustrated? You hit the goal," I said.

"Yes, but I really want to lose weight faster, so I upped it to five," she replied.

At this point, I recognized this statement as another common belief from diet culture — the idea that exercise equals weight loss, with weight loss as the only goal. There's no other reason to do it. This way of thinking harms our relationship with fitness and exercise.

It's easy to see exercise as a form of punishment — that is, if you didn't need to lose weight, you wouldn't be exercising.

Nancy and I discussed what it would be like to think of movement as a form of self-care, to be coming from a place of appreciating her body, being grateful for what it did for her every day, and treating it with kindness.

This is why one of the Fundamental Five is stated as "30 minutes of mindful movement."

BODY POSITIVITY

ANY DISCUSSION ABOUT DIET culture wouldn't be complete without addressing the body positivity movement and its take on body image.

Back in the 1960s, the Fat Acceptance movement started as an attempt to counter advocates of fat shaming. Over time, this evolved into the Body Positivity movement and expanded to include accepting and celebrating all bodies and body types, regardless of size, shape, skin tone, gender, and physical abilities.

But for some, being positive about their bodies can be a struggle. If this is the case for you, try adopting more of a body-neutral approach, where instead of focusing on what it looks like, remind yourself of all the amazing things that your body does for you and be grateful for how it supports you.

We all have flaws. No one is perfect. Why would anyone need to apologize for the size and shape of their body or any aspect of their physical appearance? The idea that they should is why body shaming and fat shaming are so harmful.

You haven't done anything wrong that you should feel guilty about or ashamed of.

JUDGMENT VS. DISCERNMENT

UNFORTUNATELY, SOME PROPONENTS OF the body positivity movement want to normalize being overweight, treating it as something that doesn't need to be addressed.

But if excess adipose tissue, such as the visceral fat in your abdominal region, increases your risk for things like heart disease, hypertension, and cancer, or if extra weight may be contributing to sleep apnea, low back pain, knee pain, and compromising your balance, then it must be addressed.

Here's the thing: If you're overweight and you don't want to lose weight, don't. No one should be judged for what they do or don't want to do with their bodies. This has nothing to do with whether you're a good person or a bad person.

There's a difference between judgment and discernment.

Discernment — what I believe is the true meaning of being accepting of your body and loving it and your life — is about looking at your life as a whole and learning what is healthy and optimal for you and the life you want.

How strong are you? What's your cardio fitness level? How flexible are you?

Yes, fitness can mitigate being overweight or obese.

But the excess weight still puts unnecessary stress on your body.

My hope for you is to find a weight that allows you to function well, perform well, be able to do what you want, feel good, and have lots of energy. And if you're listening to your body and honoring what it's telling you — using your interoception — you will find that set point that is optimal for your body.

Remember...

- Diet culture erroneously leads you to conflate the size and shape of your body with your self-worth. One has nothing to do with the other.

- Love is about who you are. Approval is about what you do.

- The judgments and opinions of others only have the power to affect how you feel about yourself if you believe them to be true.

Without the effects of diet culture, you may feel like a fish out of water at first. And there will be times when you're lulled back to the familiar.

But when you're able to see the beliefs for what they are — someone else's opinion — you now know what to do.

So, without further ado, let's get started with the Fundamental Five and how to make forming new habits a walk in the park.

Chapter 7

MAKE IT EASY AND INEVITABLE

NANCY WAS MAKING STEADY progress with her sleep habits and adding workouts into her weekly routine. Then, about eight weeks into her coaching, her husband came down with Covid, and everything turned upside down.

"I feel like all the routines and all the habits I put in place went out the window, and I have to start all over. I'm so frustrated!" she said. "I could really use some help with reframing."

"Okay, let's see," I said. "How about... this situation is helping you build resilience. You've learned a lot during the past eight weeks that you can apply going forward, so you're not really starting all over."

"Ooh... Yeah, and thinking about forming habits as building a skill helps me be more patient, too," she said.

"You're getting the hang of this reframing thing!"

APPROACH WITH A BEGINNER'S MINDSET

AS LONG AS YOU'RE alive, it's important to recognize that you can change, and you can grow.

You can develop new hobbies and learn new skills, like creating habits by design.

But this only happens when you take *imperfect* action.

I always remind folks who are trying something new that when a child is first learning to walk, do we expect them to do it perfectly?

Does falling down mean they've failed, or they're a failure?

Of course not! As a matter of fact, we know that part of learning how to walk is falling down over and over and over again.

So, when you are trying something new, experiment. Give yourself permission to fall down over and over and over again.

And just like a child learning how to walk, every time you get back up, remember you've learned something you can apply on the next attempt.

TAKING IMPERFECT ACTION

TO HELP NANCY STAY focused on learning and experimenting, I suggested she take the time every night to acknowledge her wins, both big and small, by writing them down on a card. Wins included any new learnings about what worked as well as what didn't work.

"You can put the cards in the jar I sent you," I instructed. I had labeled it "Jar of Awesome."

The next week, I asked if she had been celebrating her wins.

"To be honest, it feels silly. I don't think I should need a Jar of Awesome," she admitted.

Because she is a scientist, I knew she was familiar with the concept of negativity bias. I reminded her that our brains' priorities are safety and efficiency, leading us to focus on the negative — like the three workouts she had planned that didn't happen. That's why the Jar of Awesome was a tool she could use to shift her focus and reinterpret the outcomes in a way that would help her build momentum.

Before we wrapped things up that week, we also talked about her initial reactions to my coaching program, Joyful Eating Circles. "I didn't think it was regimented enough," she noted. "But now I understand that the reason why all the weight-loss programs I've tried before haven't work for me is because their protocols were too hard for me to sustain."

It doesn't have to be hard to lose weight. As a matter of fact, focusing on creating self-care habits is how we make it easy and inevitable.

At our session a couple of weeks later, Nancy was happy to report, "I'm getting eight hours of sleep on most nights, and my outlook throughout the day is so much better. I can tell that I focus on the negative a lot more when I'm tired, so I've been prioritizing sleep and working on ways to make sure I'm at least giving myself the opportunity to get eight hours. I used to get in bed at 10 p.m. Now, I figured out that it really helps to set an alarm to go to bed at 9:30 p.m. It's so funny that I'm setting an alarm to go to bed. Now I usually wake up before the alarm to get up goes off," she noted.

This was a true breakthrough for Nancy. The entire session had a different energy about it.

From this point forward, she had the perspective she needed to take her time building habits one by one, looking for what worked, what didn't work, and what she wanted to adjust. She fine-tuned her routine, maintaining the idea that she was already enough. She took care of herself, not because she needed to lose weight, but rather because she genuinely believed she was worth taking care of.

We focused on the habits and practices of joyful eating. And slowly but surely, she was able to identify and let go of the beliefs and rules that were based on the premise that only when you've achieved a certain size and shape will you be good enough — beliefs and rules she had previously accepted without question.

And along with letting go of those beliefs, she lost more weight.

By the time her parents visited later that summer, she had lost another five pounds without much effort because sleep and exercise were now becoming habits, making it easy for her to take consistent action.

Six months later, in early December, I received a holiday photo card from Nancy with a handwritten note. It read, "I love this photo. My heart is full. I'm beyond grateful."

AVOID OVERWHELM

IF PERFECTIONISM HAD A first cousin, it would be overwhelm.

Going forward, you're not doing overwhelm anymore. You're still going to take action, but not in the way you've done before.

To start, if you don't have the Fundamental Five self-care habits yet, these are the ones to focus on first... one at a time.

We're choosing one at a time because trying to overhaul your life or even build just two or three habits at one time — the classic all-or-nothing approach of dieting and fitness challenges — will lead to feelings of too much change and eventually overwhelm.

Simply put: If you make it hard, your brain is going to hit the brakes.

But, if you make it easy — one thing at a time — then it can be inevitable.

We're playing the long game. Believe you're going to get there, and then pick the easiest of the Fundamental Five to start.

A SIMPLE YES OR NO

WHEN CREATING A HABIT, specificity is key to making it happen.

Keeping it vague makes it much harder to discern whether or not you actually did it. Vagueness makes the situation feel more complicated, even when it isn't. And complicated can trigger thoughts of overwhelm and procrastination, those lovely thought habits that keep you from taking action.

So, make sure you take the time to define exactly what you're going to be doing.

What's the action?

When will it take place?

What items are needed?

Who else is involved, if anyone?

Then, especially when the habit still requires conscious, intentional choices, be sure to have a way to track the results.

The goal is to make it binary — a simple yes or no. Did you take the action or not?

For example, as Nancy mentioned, to create the conditions for getting eight hours of sleep, she set an alarm for 9:30 p.m. as a reminder to go to bed.

What was the action? Setting her alarm. Did she do it? Yes.

NOW IT'S YOUR TURN

WHAT HABIT DO YOU want to focus on first? How about drinking more water to stay hydrated?

Do you know how much you're drinking now?

How much more water do you want to be drinking?

How will you be able to keep track of what worked and what didn't work?

If your goal is to have one 8-ounce glass of water more than you usually have, you need to know how much you usually have, and then you need to know if you've had more.

The more specific you can get, the better.

When it comes to staying hydrated, I recommend half your body weight in ounces.

If you weigh 200 pounds, you're looking for 100 ounces. Let's say you're shooting for roughly twelve 8-ounce glasses of water.

Before coming up with your binary action, you've done some tracking, and you see that you are currently drinking five glasses of water. You decide that one more 8-ounce glass would be doable.

Now, in order to get that sixth glass of water, when are you going to drink it? What is it actually going to consist of? Will it be bottled water? Sparkling water? Hot water? Will it be part of the soup you're having for dinner?

Get as specific as possible so that, at the end of the day, you literally can say, "Yes, I did it," or "No, I didn't."

That's very different from just saying, "I want to drink more water."

You can use this technique to clarify any behavior goal, including "I want to exercise more" or "I want to move my body more" or "I want to set myself up for getting more quality sleep" or "I want to spend more time with friends and family."

FILL YOUR JAR OF AWESOME

REMEMBER THAT NEGATIVITY BIAS?

To mitigate its effects, it's important to pay attention to your wins — big and small. This is all about giving your brain evidence that what you're doing is working and that you're making it happen.

You can do this by creating your own "Jar of Awesome," where you write down your wins — both big and small — on a piece of paper and put it in a jar.

By writing it on paper, you are making it physical and giving it significance.

At a later date, you can revisit these small wins. And by re-reading them, you get double the value from the accomplishments.

If you have a tendency, as I do, to finish the day and feel like you've gotten nothing done or not enough done, write down three things you accomplished for the day on a 3 x 5 card or in a journal.

For example, if one of your goals is to lose weight, then choosing to eat a healthy breakfast or making a delicious salad for lunch is an accomplishment. For that matter, so is making time for a 7-minute workout or a 2-minute body scan to calm your nervous system if you've had a crazy, busy day.

Writing down three things will help you realize what you've accomplished in the day. You get to choose what you pay attention to, so give your brain evidence of what is working. You'll feel much better about your progress.

If you write them on a 3 x 5 card, you can put these in your "Jar of Awesome" and revisit them at the end of each week. Even the visual of watching the Jar of Awesome fill up can be a source of celebration.

The key is to make sure that you explicitly make a connection between an accomplishment and a reward.

By the way, if you're tracking your binary actions and you're on a streak, the visual can be very encouraging. Chances are, you're getting a little dopamine hit.

*You get to **choose** what you pay attention to, so give your brain **evidence** of what is **working.***

Be sure you're also tracking how you feel — your internal experience — because when you're using the visual as a reward, if and when the streak is broken, it can be very discouraging. This is when you'll want to be able to turn your attention inward.

FOLLOW THROUGH

AN EASY REWARD TO give yourself is to designate time to focus on anything you want — whether it's having dinner with a good friend, treating yourself to a blissful relaxation massage, or something mundane like cleaning your desk. Give yourself an hour to focus on that without feeling guilty that you "should" be doing something else.

Also, be diligent about ensuring the reward happens.

A client of mine achieved a very significant goal in September 2012, and she made a plan to go on a helicopter ride over the Grand Canyon. However, when February 2013 rolled around, she still hadn't done it. What message did that send to herself?

One more caveat: You will probably have self-talk about how you don't deserve the reward yet. Or that you're being silly rewarding yourself.

For instance, when I go to write down three things I've achieved for the day, there's a little voice that ALWAYS says, "This is so trivial." And yet, I know when I write down what I have done for the day, I feel better.

So, make a plan for celebrating the small victories, too.

It's very easy to find reasons not to celebrate them, but small wins build confidence and momentum and are part of enjoying the journey.

I suggest setting aside some time today (put a calendar reminder on your phone) to plan some rewards for activities you're doing now. Once you've done that, be sure to follow through on rewarding yourself when you've done the tasks.

MAKE IT A WALK IN THE PARK

ANOTHER ONE OF MY clients, Audrey, came to me with a very familiar wish. She had heard a meditation practice has a lot of benefits, including stress relief, more focus, and becoming an observer of your thoughts. We had been working on identifying her triggers around emotional eating, so becoming more aware of her thoughts was something she was working on.

She also had a very specific goal: to meditate 20 minutes a day. She had read somewhere that 20 minutes a day was ideal.

And on the few occasions she had been able to meditate in a yoga class, she noticed how much better she felt and how much more focused she was.

I heartily agreed it was a great goal to aim for, but as soon as I asked a follow-up question, "What time of day do you want to do this?

She said, "I don't really have time to meditate 20 minutes a day, but if I could fit some meditation in before the twins wake up, that would be great."

"Could you do 10 minutes?" I asked. "Would that be easier?" She responded, "Oh, yeah. Definitely."

I followed up. "On a scale of 1 to 10, where 1 is very difficult, and 10 is a walk in the park, how would you rate this?"

"Somewhere around a 7 or 8?" she answered.

"Hmm.... what makes it a 7 or 8 instead of a 6?" I asked.

"Well, since my plan is to do it in the morning before the twins wake up, I just need to wake up a few minutes before they do," she replied.

"What would make it a 9 or 10?" I continued.

"If it was less than 5 minutes," she answered.

"What would make it a 10?" I asked.

"I believe I could do 2 minutes every morning before the twins wake up," she said.

"How about we try that for a couple of weeks and then add slowly over time?" I suggested.

"That works for me," Audrey replied cheerily.

"Okay, let's see what happens," I said.

When I checked in with her a week later, she said, "I'm so proud of myself. I meditated for two minutes every day this past week. And..." She had a big grin on her face as she continued, "On the one morning I chose to sleep in, instead of being derailed, I found two minutes between Zoom calls."

A few weeks later, she reported, "I feel so good. Two minutes feels like a piece of cake. I think I'll try 5 minutes."

Six months later, she was up to 15 minutes twice a day.

HAVE A PLAN B

SPEAKING OF IMPERFECT ACTION, how often does your day go perfectly as planned?

If you spend some time thinking about and anticipating what might get in the way of making IT happen, you'll be able to come up with a Plan B or C or D.

For Audrey, experimenting was key to discovering how to make her new habits stick. Having already worked with me for six months, she came up with a Plan B on her own for the mornings she chose to sleep in.

You can do this too. By experimenting, you'll learn if something worked or didn't, or if it worked, but only in certain kinds of situations.

The point is this. You want to approach new tasks with the mindset, "Let me try this and see what happens."

Quite frankly, if you knew what the outcome would be, it wouldn't be an experiment.

So, give yourself permission to fail. Look for the lesson.

That's how you grow.

YOU GOT THIS

FREQUENCY AND REPETITION HELP to build momentum.

With daily habits, the cumulative benefits and compounding effect also mean you'll be able to notice changes happening more quickly and adjust the trajectory more significantly over time.

That's why I recommend starting with one of the Fundamental Five.

You'll get a bigger bang for your buck, as the impact of daily habits is more significant than those done weekly, monthly, quarterly, or annually.

So, the next time you're looking at building a habit or learning a new skill, when something seems like it's too hard...

Think about it like this: What's the smallest version of it you're confident you can do?

Or try asking yourself, "How can I make it fun?"

If your goal is to build a habit of 30 minutes of mindful movement, and a 30-minute HIIT class feels like torture right now, how about:

A 30-minute walk or stretching class?

Or three 10-minute walks?

Or just one flight of stairs?

Or a few more steps because you parked a little further from the front door of the grocery store?

Because it all counts! It all moves you a little closer to your goal.

The alternative is doing nothing because you talk yourself out of going back to the HIIT class that was too hard at this time.

This thought process applies not just to movement but also to any habit or skill you're developing.

Can you find a way to drink just one more glass?

Or eat one more serving of green leafy vegetables?

Or go to bed 15 minutes earlier?

Think back to our scale of 1 to 10, where 10 is a walk in the park. If you're not rating whatever version of that habit you've chosen as 9 or 10, you'll want to shrink down the task until you're confident in your ability to make it happen.

Give your brain evidence that you can do it by watching yourself doing it, build self-efficacy and confidence, pay attention to what works, and build on these.

Remember...

- The road to success is paved with failures and lessons.

- Life happens, so make a plan B.

- Celebrate your wins — big and small.

- Give your brain evidence that you have what it takes.

- Make it easy, so it can become inevitable.

And, as you know, easy is subjective. What's easy for you may be extremely difficult for someone else, and vice versa.

So, if you catch yourself playing the comparison game, remind yourself that this is about running your own race.

Chapter 8

CREATE THE LIFE YOU WANT

"Today is my new favorite day."— *Winnie The Pooh*

TO CELEBRATE OUR 10TH anniversary, my partner, Matt, and I had dinner at the Ritz Carlton in Half Moon Bay, California. It's a beautiful hotel sitting high above the beach with a panoramic view of the Pacific Ocean.

When it came time for dessert, we did our usual. I looked at the menu and spotted an apple crumble à la mode that sounded tasty.

"I'll just have a bite or two," Matt said.

Mind you, one of his bites is equivalent to three of mine.

We usually share a dessert since Matt doesn't have much of a sweet tooth, and I usually just want to end dinner with something sweet on my palate. More often than not, we don't finish it.

So, we ordered two coffees and the one dessert.

When the waiter came back, he placed the white ramekin with the apple crumble and ice cream in front of me, along with two forks, two big spoons, and our two coffees. The presentation was lovely.

We thanked him, and as I pushed the dessert to the center of the table, we each picked up a spoon.

As I took the first bite, I felt my taste buds doing a happy dance. *It was easily the best apple crumble I'd ever had.*

The apple had just the right amount of chew — not too soft — and was plenty warm with a hint of cinnamon and the coolness of the vanilla ice cream. What made it special was the blueberries they had added.

It was so good; I didn't want to share.

Of course, just as that thought crossed my mind, I watched Matt scoop up one of his big bites.

"It's okay, Amy," I said to myself. "It's just dessert," as I took a sip of coffee.

And then, with alarm and dismay, I watched him scoop up another bite.

Seriously, in that moment, I was about to reach across the table to stab his hand until I realized I was clutching a spoon, not a fork.

"Two of his bites is half of the dessert," I thought to myself.

If you ever want to know what it feels like to be in a state of scarcity, I'm describing it.

And one of the thoughts I had was that Matt was depriving me of something I wanted.

I considered my options. I could yank his spoon away from him, I could block his access to the dessert with my arm, or I could just start crying.

"Amy, you're being silly," I tried to calm myself.

And then it came to me.

I looked at Matt and said, "If we finish this, and I still want more, I'm ordering another one."

"So that's why you were glaring at me. You must really like it," he said, smiling.

Yep, it's true. I'm not some super-evolved being. I have cravings, too.

It's our common humanity. We all experience feelings of scarcity or guilt or discouragement around food and excess fat, especially around our midsections.

But instead of letting our unexamined thoughts — the stampeding elephant — control us, we can learn how to recognize when the thoughts are triggering us and harness the elephant's power.

ONE PIECE AT A TIME

AT THIS POINT, YOU probably have a list of habits that your future self will be practicing every day. You can picture it in your mind's eye.

And when you become aware of limiting beliefs and the interpretations that follow, you'll be able to insert a pause and reinterpret them. The actions you take, with practice and consistency, will create the conditions that make the outcomes you desire easy and inevitable.

That's the goal: mastery of a skillset — what you can control.

You'll be putting pieces in place, one at a time, like a jigsaw puzzle.

And if you know anything about jigsaw puzzles, you know that you want to create the frame first. Those edge pieces are easy to find. There aren't very many of them compared to the total number of pieces, and when you've put them in place, they provide structure.

When it comes to lasting weight loss and rediscovering joyful eating, the four pillars of the Joyful Eating Framework are the corners, and the Fundamental Five are your edge pieces.

The practices that stem from the four pillars — acceptance, boundaries, compassion, interoceptive fidelity, and perceptual positioning — will form the finished puzzle that will be your version of Joyful Eating in action.

THE TENSION OF OPPOSITES

IF YOU HAVE A history of dieting, your brain has lots of evidence that weight loss, especially lasting weight loss, is hard.

But again, it doesn't have to be. It can be easy.

It depends on the approach.

I know this is counterintuitive.

*If you know anything about **jigsaw puzzles**, you know that you want to **create the frame** first.*

So, if you're on the fence about trying again, I'd like you to try this exercise.

You're going to evaluate the pros and cons of changing versus staying the same.

If you're inclined to stay where you are, it's probably because you're thinking about the pros of staying the same. It's the devil you know. And you get to stay in your comfort zone.

You're also dwelling on the cons of changing — that is, fear, uncertainty, and doubt.

What kinds of fears?

Perhaps the most common one is fear of the outcome — like losing the weight only to gain it back, which is usually interpreted as failure. (But now you know better.)

You might also fear the process.

Maybe you've read somewhere that, to eat healthier, you need to cook your meals at home, and that idea worries you because you don't know how to cook. Or maybe you want to start strength training, but you have no idea what exercises to do, and you're afraid you're going to wind up hurting yourself.

And then there's the fear of loss. A lot of times, when it comes to eating healthier, a lot of folks are afraid they won't be able to socialize with their friends anymore, especially when it involves food and alcohol.

Or you could fear how the change will impact an intimate relationship, especially if you've suffered trauma and have been using the extra weight as a form of protection.

Or perhaps you haven't been able to find the right relationship for yourself, and, up until this point, you've been able to blame it on your weight. However, in the back of your mind, you've always feared that the problem is you, that you're broken beyond repair.

But remember, just because you have the thought, that doesn't make it true. The previous examples show that there's not much tension when you're looking at the pros of staying the same and the cons of changing. Staying the same seems like a much smaller risk. The payoff for change doesn't seem worth it.

To overcome this perception, do this instead: Take a piece of paper and write the change you're contemplating at the top. On the left side, list all the cons of staying the same, like all the pain you've experienced with dieting. Then, on the right side, list all the pros of changing, like all the benefits of Joyful Eating.

Focus on creating tension. Make the cons of not changing and the pros of changing as far apart in positive and negative emotion as possible.

And, when it comes to the tension of opposites, if you're wondering which side will win, in the words of the indomitable Morrie Schwartz:

"Love wins. Love always wins."[13]

YOUR JOURNEY

LIKE HAPPINESS, JOYFUL EATING isn't a destination. It's a journey. It's something I hope you get to experience each and every day.

To start, you just need to do one more thing.

Make a decision.

Make a decision right now to take one small step forward to take better care of yourself.

Make it an easy one.

It could be to ask a better question. Or...

Go for a walk.

Call a friend.

Breathe deeply.

Start journaling.

Say no, and mean it.

Ask for what you want.

Give yourself permission.

Say yes more often.

There are so many different small steps you can take.

Because you deserve all the delicious goodness each one brings.

Speaking of delicious, true to form, Matt only took two bites of the dessert. I slowly savored my small bites. And by the time I took my last bite, I felt completely content.

THIS MOMENT

TODAY IS A GIFT.

That's why it's called the present.

You have the power to create the life you want by taking action right now. This very moment.

Postscript

*"No act of kindness, no matter
how small, is ever wasted."* — Aesop

I HOPE YOU'VE FOUND this book helpful and that you've already started building one of the Fundamental Five using the Easy and Inevitable method.

I'd love to know which habit you chose to focus on first, if you have thoughts that are getting in the way, what other challenges you have encountered, and how I may be of assistance in your journey to Joyful Eating. You can email me at feedback@amylangcoaching.com. I read every email personally, and I would love to hear from you. Perhaps, we'll even get a chance to work together someday soon.

One Last Thing... According to research, helping others is associated with greater health, happiness, and longevity.[14]

It's been called the "helper's high."

And you have an opportunity here to do just that.

If you've found this book helpful, please share what you've learned. You can do so by leaving a detailed review of the book.

It will help others who could benefit from it make the decision to get it, read it, and apply what they've learned.

Thank you for your time and attention. It's been an honor and a privilege to share my journey with you.

Save room for dessert. ♥

About the Author

AMY LANG IS A master health coach, certified personal trainer, and host of the *Happy & Healthy with Amy* podcast. She helps people who want to achieve lasting weight loss create the self-care habits that make their goal easy and inevitable.

After a decade in the high-tech industry, working at companies like Netscape, Oracle, and Yahoo, Amy decided to take a chance on herself and pursue her lifelong passion: real healthcare.

She's been in the health and fitness industry since 2003: first, as the owner of Pacific Heights Health Club in San Francisco, where she and her team helped thousands of clients achieve their health and fitness goals, and then, as the founder of Moxie Club, an online coaching business she started in December 2019, where her reach has expanded across the US, as well as Canada, Australia, and Western Europe.

When she's not coaching, Amy enjoys traveling, playing tennis, eating roast crab, and spending time with her partner, Matt, and her Bernedoodle puppy, Moxie!

For information on her coaching services, speaking engagements, and digital courses, and for more information on all aspects of forming habits and a healthy lifestyle, including free workshops, live events, and the Joyful Eating Toolkit, visit **AmyLangCoaching.com.**

Endnotes

1 *The Dukes of Hazzard*, season 3, episode 9, "The Great
   Santa Claus Chase," directed by Denver Pyle, aired
   December 19, 1980, CBS.
2 Matthew Budd, M.D. and Larry Rothstein, Ed.D., *You Are
   What You Say* (New York: Three Rivers Press, 2000), page 125.
3 Anne Craig, "Discovery of 'thought worms' opens
   window to the mind," *Queen's Gazette*, July 13,
   2020, https://www.queensu.ca/gazette/stories/
   discovery-thought-worms-opens-window-mind.
4 Cambridge Dictionary Online, s.v. "habit" (n), accessed
   May 7, 2023, https://dictionary.cambridge.org/us/
   dictionary/english/habit.
5 Evelyn Tribole and Elyse Resch, *Intuitive Eating* (New
   York: St. Martin's Publishing Group, 2020), page 46.
6 *Saturday Night Live*, season 42, episode 23, "Weekend
   Update Summer Edition, directed by Don Roy King,
   written by Tina Fey, Colin Jost, and Michael Che,
   featuring Tina Fey, aired August 17, 2017, NBC.
7 Jonathan Haidt, *The Happiness Hypothesis*, (New York:
   Basic Books, 2005), page 17.
8 Marianne Cumella Reddan, Tor Dessart Wager, Daniela
   Schiller, "Attenuating Neural Threat Expression with
   Imagination," *Neuron*, 100, no. 4 (November 21, 2018),
   994-1005, https://doi.org/10.1016/j.neuron.2018.10.047.

9   Abraham Maslow, "A Theory of Human Motivation," *Psychological Review* (1943), 50(4), 370–396. https://doi.org/10.1037/h0054346

10 Robert Waldinger and Marc Schulz, *The Good Life* (New York: Simon & Schuster, 2023).

11 Lauri Nummenmaa, Enrico Glerean, Riitta Hari, and Jari K. Hietanen, "Bodily Maps of Emotions," *Psychological and Cognitive Sciences* 111, no. 2. (December 30, 2013): 646–651, https://www.pnas.org/doi/full/10.1073/pnas.1321664111.

12 Expert Market Research, *Global Weight Loss and Weight Management Diet Market Share, Size, Growth, Analysis, Forecast,* accessed August 12, 2023, https://www.expertmarketresearch.com/reports/weight-loss-and-weight-management-diet-market.

13 Mitch Albom, *Tuesdays with Morrie* (New York: Doubleday, 1997), p 40.

14 Stephen G. Post, *The Hidden Gifts of Helping* (San Francisco: Jossey-Bass, 2011).